New Perspectives on Contraception

by

Donald DeMarco, Ph.D.

ISBN 0-9669777-1-8

Published by
One More Soul
616 Five Oaks Avenue
Dayton, Ohio 45406

Cover art by René Magritte, "The Lovers," 1928.
© 1999. C. Herscovici, Brussles/Artists Rights Society (ARS), New York

Some chapters of *New Perspectives on Contraception* have appeared, in variously modified forms, in the following journals: *Homiletic & Pastoral Review, The New Oxford Review, Culture Wars, Catholic Faith, Social Justice Review, Child & Family Quarterly,* and *Bulletin of the Ovulation Method Research and Reference Centre of Australia.*

Printed by
St. Martin de Porres Lay Dominican Community
New Hope KY 40052

*This book is proudly dedicated to
my daughter, Jocelyn,
who was born in 1968, and
my son-in-law, Leo,
who became husband and wife
in July of 1998 on the
30th Anniversary of*
Humanae Vitae.

Table of Contents

Foreword

We have known Dr. Donald De Marco for several years now and soon learned to respect and admire him, since we first met him and listened to him at a Conference in Vancouver, Canada. Subsequently he came to Australia on a successful Lecture Tour when he kindly consented to speak to some of our natural family planning teachers and various youth groups who were much edified by what he had to say. He is a great philosopher who fortunately possesses the ability to explain philosophy clearly.

The latest publication **New Perspectives on Contraception** is an excellent book. It is the product of observation of contraceptive practises over almost 40 years and exhibits deep insight into their physical, philosophical and spiritual effects upon the world. He writes truly when he tells us that courage, love, knowledge all go together to remedy the devastation of the "Culture of Death".

At the beginning he introduces a most appropriate quotation from St. Thomas Aquinas, "The greatest kindness one can render to any man consists in leading him to truth". There are many other quotations and commentaries which show his wide scholarship, for example, from Pope John Paul II's **Evangelium Vitae** and Pope Paul VI's **Humanae Vitae**. The physical complications of various modern contraceptive techniques are well documented, and the statistics are supplied with good references. He contrasts those problems with the benefits which flow from the use of natural family planning in marriage, benefits not only to health but also to married love.

We agree with all that Donald has to say in what is an excellent summary of the battle between good and evil in modern times, where the battlefield has been over the graves of millions of helpless babies, conceived lovelessly and ruthlessly destroyed, where the casualties have been marriages and other relationships fragmented by contraception, where the only answers that could have solved the problems of these unhappy people were Truth and Love.

It is hoped that this book will find a wide distribution. It could be extremely helpful to priests, marriage counsellors, senior High School students and young adults contemplating marriage.

Evelyn L. Billings   John J. Billings

Acknowledgement

I am most grateful to many people in the field of contraceptive and natural family planning research for their knowledge, encouragement, and personal example. While I cannot mention by name everyone to whom I am indebted, I would like to take this opportunity to thank a few who have truly been giants in the field: Drs. John and Lyn Billings, the late Dr. Herb Ratner, John and Kathi Hamlon, Judie Brown, John and Sheila Kippley, Professors Janet E. Smith and William E. May, Reverends Paul Marx, OSB and Joseph Hattie, OMI, Drs. Hanna Klaus, Tom W. Hilgers, Chris Kahlenborn, and Paul Byrne. And finally to William Lindahl, PhD, for his careful and competent reading and critique of the entire manuscript.

I am also indebted to my son, Don, Jr., for his patience in cheerfully and frequently serving as my computer guide and glitch repairman.

Above all, I am happy to express my debt of gratitude to Steve Koob, Director of One More Soul, who has been the prime mover, catalyst, and executor extraordinaire for this project. It can truly be said that without his encouragement and inspiration, *New Perspectives on Contraception* would never have gotten started.

Donald DeMarco
Kitchener, Ontario
July 25, 1998 — **The 30th Anniversary of** *Humanae Vitae*

*"The greatest kindness one
can render to any man
consists in leading
him to truth."*

. . . Thomas Aquinas

Contraception and God's Plan

I was teaching an introductory philosophy course to a class of first-year university students. We were discussing Plato's celebrated analogy of the Cave. One of the essential, but problematic tasks a philosophy teacher inherits is to explore with students the possibility that, despite whatever high opinion they might have of themselves, they may very well be in the dark about certain things. I had good reason to believe that my students, by and large, were in the dark about contraception. How does a teacher nudge his students toward the light on this important issue which most of them assume has been settled for all time?

University students want to be progressive and up-to-date. They do not want to parrot their parents' opinions or be tied in any way to the past. But at the same time, they do not want to be conditioned by their environment. They want to be simultaneously trendy and independent. Since 85% of their information, according to experts, comes from a meretricious Mass Media, however, this is a most difficult combination for them to realize.

According to Plato's analogy of the Cave, human beings are content with a world of shadows or illusions. They are blissfully unaware that they are deprived of the light that illuminates reality. The great task of education, for Plato, is to lead students from illusion to reality. Students, however, underestimate the breadth and depth of Plato's Cave. They assume that they have escaped the Cave because they have escaped the past. What they do not realize is that the Cave is a maze of many rooms. One may escape Chamber A and find oneself not out of the Cave, but solidly entrenched in Chamber B.

A philosophy teacher would render his students a grave disservice if he convinced them that they had fled the Cave when they had only migrated from one room to another. Surely a teacher should be kind, and, as Saint Thomas Aquinas writes, "The greatest kindness one can render to any man consists in leading him from error to truth."[1] There must be at least one critical instance, I thought, when all my students must oppose the use of contraception. Therefore, the question I posed to them was this: "How many of you are not op-posed to your parents' use of contraception at the time you were conceived?" Perhaps naively, I expected that all of them, happy to exist, would be pleased that their parents did not contracept them, thereby preventing them from coming into being. I was unduly opti-mistic. One student took pains to explain to me (since I, it seemed, was the one who occupied the Cave) that it was all simply a matter of choice and that he was perfectly willing to accept whatever choice his parents might have made.

This was a wing in Plato's labyrinth that I should have antici-pated. Today's society is in love with "choice", even to the point, at times, when some individuals prefer another's choice to their own existence. This may seem to be a gesture of heroic altruism, but, I thought, in upholding an abstract choice over one's own concrete ex-istence, one exhibits a curious preference for shadow over substance. Besides, if we were to love our neighbor as we love ourselves, a minimal expression of self-love would be to affirm our own exist-ence. Can we not be grateful that our parents made, not any choice, but the noncontraceptive choice that led to our existence? From the parental point of view, would they not be pleased that their noncontraceptive intercourse produced offspring who lived, loved, developed, and ultimately populated my classroom as first-year seekers of philosophical wisdom?

What this line of discussion comes to has far-reaching implica-tions. Now that contraception is largely accepted in contemporary society, and now that individuals (married or not) have the "choice" as to whether their union will or will not produce offspring, does this mean that we can no longer see ourselves as part of God's Plan? Given the current situation, is it still possible for any of us to relate our existence to a divine plan that imbues our life with a transcen-dent meaning? Are we creatures who are part of God's plan? Or are we merely creatures of human choice? Are we children of God? Or children of chance? We can be grateful to God for our existence be-cause God is a person. But we can not be grateful to choice, espe-cially since, in respecting choice, we must have equal respect for the contraceptive choice that would have prevented our coming to be.

Plato, who had much more affection for reality than illusion, taught that real love expresses itself by the desire to generate what is beautiful, in the body or the soul: "The bodies and souls of all hu-man beings are alike pregnant with their future progeny, and when we arrive at a certain age, our nature impels us to bring forth and propagate." G. K. Chesterton talked about the irrepressible desire he had to thank someone for the gift of life. When we think of ourselves as existing between love and gratitude, it is easy for us to think that our life has meaning and that in some profound and mysterious way, it is part of a plan, one that may, in fact, begin in the mind and heart of God.

Choice and *plan* are compatible with each other, but only insofar as choice submits to plan. When choice is made into an ideology, however, with its unremitting emphasis on freedom, it becomes completely divorced from plan, and consequently, from order, coherence, and direction. If there is to be any discernible meaning in life, choice must submit to plan.

Imagine twenty people trying to watch a video, each one operating a hand-held remote control unit that allows him to pause, fast-forward, or rewind the film at will. Each person is free to exercise his choice as he sees fit and does so with no regard whatsoever for anyone else's viewing interest. The result is predictable chaos. No one sees the movie the way it was originally intended to be seen. Uncoordinated choice makes it impossible for anyone to appreciate the plan of the movie. Random choices effectively obliterate any observable semblance of order. If people want to enjoy their video, they must choose to limit their collective use of the remotes. Ironically, in multiplying choices, the one choice that is sacrificed is the choice to watch the movie.

God has a plan for us, but our often willful and licentious exercise of choice can easily obscure it (though it cannot obliterate it). Contraception breeds a mentality of individualism that severs choice from any semblance of a plan. The absence of any discernible plan leads to a sense of disorder. The perception today is that there is so much disorder in the world that despair seems to be more realistic than belief in some over-arching Plan. Yet this mentality is characteristic of Plato's cave dweller. It is possible to rediscover a sense of God's Plan for human beings. In order to follow this road to discovery, which leads out of the Cave, one must assume the mentality not of the contraceptivist, but of the detective. Philosophers and sleuths have often been compared with each other since they are both trying to solve a mystery by starting from effects and carefully, and logically proceeding toward finding the cause. The first place to begin our detective work is by studying the *Natural Law*.

The Natural Law

The *natural law* is not the same thing as the *laws of nature*. The former has a moral dimension, the latter does not. One is an inclination or disposition, the other is a demonstrable fact. The Ancients referred to the natural law as the *unwritten law* and held that it was imprinted on the hearts of men. In Sophocles' great drama, *Antigone*, the heroine pleaded that her brother should be given a dignified burial on the basis of this natural law that is engraved on the hearts of all men. Galileo referred to the laws of nature when he wrote about the Book of Nature which is written in the language of mathematics. These laws represent the intelligibility of nature and provide the basis for empirical sciences such as physics, chemistry, and biology.

At the same time, though distinct, the natural law is not separate from the laws of nature. In fact, it incorporates it. Man grows and ages. This is a fact of biology, one that flows from the laws of man's nature. But there is no such law of his nature that impels him to become more moral, that is to say, a better or more virtuous human being. He must choose freely to be moral; but biological growth belongs, fundamentally, not to the order of freedom and morality, as does the natural law, but to the realm of necessity and the laws of nature (which are interpreted by the physical sciences).

Contraception itself could not have been developed and improved without considerable knowledge of the sciences, especially chemistry and biology. It presents a moral problem not because it emerges from a knowledge of the laws of nature, but because it is contrary to the natural law. Many critics have stated that because the Catholic Church opposes contraception, she must also oppose science and scientific progress. Nothing could be further from the truth. The Church does not oppose knowledge of the laws of nature, but she does oppose application of that knowledge when it is contrary to the natural law, which inclines man to what is good for him as a whole in the pursuit of his destiny.

Knowledge of the laws of nature help man to understand who he is, but they are not sufficient to advise him about how he should live. Man is not merely an animal; nor is he a being whose full meaning reveals itself to the scientist. He has a spiritual dimension that transcends the world of science (the laws of nature). He has an inborn sense of what he ought to do, and this is the natural law that is imprinted on his heart. Moreover, in doing what he ought to do, he directs his life toward its fullness which he experiences, as Aristotle contends, in the form of personal happiness.

There is a philosophy of individualism that honors no other law than will or freedom. This philosophy owes much to the 18th century philosopher Jean-Jacques Rousseau who advised that one should "obey only himself." The problem with obeying only oneself, however, despite its enormous popularity in the contemporary world, is that it alienates the person from the natural law that embraces his physical as well as his spiritual nature. It represents a mode of living that has lost its anchor in nature. It is a philosophy based on something as shadowy and unreliable as whim and illusion. Moreover, it does not represent a philosophy that one could share with others in the interest of working together for a common good.

The natural law is a realistic and reliable basis on which we can understand who we are and how we are to act. We are often vain and selfish. The natural law brings us back to reality. Moreover, the natural law is a reflection of God's eternal law. We begin to discern God's Plan, however dimly, when we begin to appreciate the natural law. For this reason, the great philosophers of antiquity understood that since nature comes from God, the natural law is founded in Creative Wisdom itself. We honor God by honoring the nature He created.

Marriage, because it is essentially involved with nature, love, procreation, and community, places husband and wife in a particularly advantageous position to appreciate God's Plan. Pope Paul VI has stated that "God the Creator wisely and providentially established marriage with the intent that he might achieve His own design to love through Men" (*Humanae vitae*, sec.8). But the use of contraception, which separates sexual union from procreation, represents an act that withdraws from nature and the natural law, thereby isolating the partners from that which gives marriage its proper direction. It is an act that can make God's Plan increasingly difficult to see. "What is contraception," asks John Kippley, "except the studied effort to take apart what God has put together?"[2] Typical of a growing number of medical doctors, Kim Anthony Hardey, who is a Board Certified Obstetrician/Gynecologist in Lafayette, Louisiana, has made the following statement: "In 1993, I became convinced that artificial contraception was not part of God's Plan. I was also convinced that providing or using artificial contraception was a serious offense against God, in which I no longer could participate. I left my contraceptive practice . . .to set up a new practice that has been totally free of any contraception or sterilization."[3]

Withdrawing from nature and suppressing the natural law in one's heart can prove calamitous. Contraception can often be the gateway to such calamity. By adopting contraception, one takes an important step toward adopting a contraceptive philosophy that replaces living by the natural law with living by one's own law of freedom. The disorder of contraception may not be evident to everyone, but the disorders it invites — sterilization, abortion, experimental reproductive technologies, divorce, *etc.* — become increasingly evident to the point of becoming undeniable.

Philosopher-theologian Germain Grisez reports a letter he received in which a woman highlights the tragic life of her sister. The sister left the Church while attending Harvard's business school. While she pursued her ten-year career she had several affairs and abortions. When she quit work to marry and have children, she encountered a complicated fertility problem. She sought to have a child through *in vitro* fertilization using donor semen, but the first attempt failed. One 'spare' embryo was frozen. Before a second attempt was made, her husband left her for his secretary. Sensing she had no reason to live, she committed suicide. The woman wants to know about the morality of becoming a surrogate gestator for her sister's frozen embryo.[4]

The late Herbert Ratner, a distinguished public health physician, editor, and international lecturer, was fond of stating that God always forgives, man sometimes forgives, and nature never forgives. We disregard the laws of nature and the natural law at great personal peril. One might expect that the subject of the tragic case outlined above would, if she could live her life over again, live it in a way that expressed more respect for nature and less for "doing one's own thing." Perspective can be, like hindsight, 20-20. How can we maintain the right perspective when the pressures and temptations of the moment can be so powerful that they block out everything else? In this regard, the art of storytelling can be most helpful. A good story offers the advantage of placing past, present, and future into perspective in order to show that the greater meaning of the moment lies in how well it serves the unfolding of a plan. Both life and the natural law fully reveal themselves on the horizon of time.

Perspective

Manipulating time and the events that transpire in time in order to illustrate the moral significance and the drama of human life has been used with great success. Consider, for example, Charles Dickens' classic *Christmas Carol* or Frank Capra's immensely popular film, *It's a Wonderful Life*. Consider, also, three extremely successful Hollywood films made in three consecutive years, from 1984-86, in which time is altered to illustrate the drama and moral significance of procreation. In each of these movies, the heroes or heroines go back to the past where they must make sacrifices and overcome obstacles in order to assure that certain lives, destined to be conceived, will indeed be conceived.

In the 1984 film, *The Terminator*, Arnold Schwarzenegger plays the role of a virtually indestructible cyborg who is sent back in time from the year 2029 to assassinate a woman who is destined to give birth to a great and noble revolutionary leader. Another man, Reese, also returns from the future in order to father this child. Reese has the privilege of knowing his son in the future, and his love for him is so great that he is willing to face any danger in order to conceive him. Once he completes his task as conceptor, he willingly sacrifices his life to save his child.

In *Back to the Future* (1985), Michael J. Fox plays a character who travels 30 years back in time to his parents' past high school days where he must play cupid to ensure that two people who are to become his parents, marry each other. The young man's very existence is at stake, for if his prospective parents do not get together, he will never be conceived.

Kathleen Turner plays the lead in the 1986 movie, *Peggy Sue Got Married*, in which she attends her twenty-fifth high school reunion, passes out, and when she comes to, is twenty-seven years younger. Now a high-school teenager, with the mind and memory of a forty-two year old woman, she is faced with an agonizing decision. Should she marry her high-school beau, knowing that he will cheat on her and that her marriage will result in separation and possibly divorce? But her love for the two children they will conceive makes all of her heartache seem worthwhile and gives her sufficient motivation to marry this man a second time.

When married people practice contraception, it is usually because the child they want to avoid at the time is judged to represent more difficulties than they are prepared to assume. This is perhaps the sensible choice, but certainly not the dramatic one. Most people seem to be fearful of dramatic uncertainty and try to orchestrate their lives accordingly. Security and predictability is what they prefer. Drama is for fiction, not for "real life."

A story, needless to say, is as dull as dishwater if it has no drama. But the moral significance of a good story, like the three outlined above, is to remind us that by clinging to security, we deny ourselves the chance of living out the story we are destined to live, one that is much more personally fulfilling. In a word, our desire for security can *contracept* our experience of authenticity. We should not relegate good stories to the realm of mere entertainment. We should be able to profit from them on a moral level. A good story suggests to us that there is a noble plan we are all destined to realize, one that is fraught with difficulties and uncertainties, but infinitely more enriching than the relatively colorless lives we often select.

The three aforementioned stories, by imaginatively altering the natural sequence of time, help us to be more appreciative of the wholeness of life. They remind us how each moment in the present, which soon becomes part of the past, has a vital bearing on the future. Contraception rests on a philosophy of life that assigns exaggerated importance to the difficulties of the moment and de-emphasizes the significance of everything else on the time spectrum. The stories give us perspective, and teach us that by overcoming difficulties we can realize a higher plan.

Psychiatrist Viktor Frankl is the founder of the school of *logotherapy*, which has been hailed as the Third Viennese School of Psychotherapy. Logotherapy is a technique of healing people by helping them to find the meaning of their lives. It is Frankl's firm conviction that man is more profoundly a meaning-oriented being than a comfort or pleasure seeking being. "Man can endure any *how*," he writes, "as long as he has a *why*." He warns, then, that any absence of tension in one's life can be as dangerous to one's mental health as too much tension.[5]

One aspect of the logotherapy technique is to invite patients to see their lives in perspective, that is, to transcend the moment and view life as a whole. When they do this, they begin to see that suffering and uncertainty are not necessarily negative factors that should always be avoided, but can actually contribute to an overall sense of life's meaning. Suffering may indeed be needed so that this higher meaning can be realized.

Logotherapy provides perspective and it assists people in overcoming their fear of the future. Because of this, it can be a great help in counteracting a contraceptive philosophy of life. The imaginative perspective that both logotherapy and good storytelling provide have much in common with the natural law. All three emphasize that meaning, authenticity, and personal fulfillment often require taking the higher road, one that is strewn with obstacles, hazards, and difficulties. Helpful as they may be, however, they still require some measure of faith, since few if any of us can read the future.

Faith

Kierkegaard alluded to a fundamental dilemma in human existence when he pointed out that we know backwards but must live forwards. Everything we know is about that which has already taken place. The future, by contrast, seems to be a leap into darkness. Knowledge of history is not a basis for predicting the future. Heading into tomorrow by looking through a rear-view window is not a reliable way of traveling.

People resist faith. But what they often replace it with is fear. Two teenagers, engaged to each other, approached a medical doctor and requested that he sterilize both of them. The doctor declined, since he thought they were too young to make such an important and irreversible decision. But he was curious about what both of them wanted to be sterilized. Would it not be sufficient to sterilize just one? They explained to him, rather tersely, that they did not trust each other. They wanted to be married to each other, retain their double income, and remain open to the possibility of engaging in extra-marital affairs. They were, in their own minds, thoroughly open and totally liberated. But could a more penetrating assessment of their relationship be that it is *faithless*?

Faithlessness is akin to lovelessness. It is not in the nature of love to be sterile. There is no such thing as a sterile love. Love is, by virtue of its own inner essence, creative. It is naturally hope-filled and full of faith. It cannot help but imagine a brighter tomorrow.

The noted economist, Lewis Lehrman was once criticized by a woman for the apparent irresponsibility he exhibited in siring five children. They will consume "precious natural resources," she protested. "But Madam," he retorted, "don't you understand? Those children themselves, are our most precious natural resources." Children are not the problem; not to have them is not the solution. Thomas Malthus' great anxiety about population was linked not only to his rejection of Providence, but to his unexplainable reduction of human beings to mouths without minds. He saw human beings, as many do today, not as contributors but only as consumers.

The teenage couple who rejected progeny and distrusted each other were actually imposing a curse upon themselves without realizing it. In Shakespeare's *King Lear*, Goneril's display of ingratitude fills her father with such blinding rage that he invokes the ultimate curse on her:

Hear, nature, hear; dear goddess,
Suspend thy purpose, if thou didst intend
To make this creature fruitful:
Into her womb convey sterility:
Dry up in her the organs of increase.
And from her derogate body
A babe to honour her!

Planned Parenthood is an organization that believes, almost religiously, we might say, in planning. Its unwavering commitment to and confidence in contraception, as history has shown, is ample testimony for this claim. But its faith is in its plan, and we all know what often happens to the best laid schemes of mice and men. True faith transcends planning. To plan without faith is, as Kierkegaard pointed out, like trying to live life backwards. We cannot plan for things that are more wonderful than we could imagine, or even for pleasant surprises. The natural plan should make room for the supernatural intervention. "There is no road has not a star above it," wrote the American essayist, Ralph Waldo Emerson. This exquisite phrase symbolizes the blending of plan with faith, the natural with the supernatural, the earthly with the Divine. Marriage, as Genesis proclaims, is of Godly origin. It is not likely that God would abandon what he instituted to the unreliable institutions of human planning.

God's Plan has both natural and mysterious components. It requires us to exercise our intelligence and our imagination as well as our faith. Saint Thomas Aquinas was once asked how he could justify the great confidence he had in what he wrote. He answered that it was because he learned from two primary sources that could not lie: nature and Scripture. Given the fact that a high percentage of our information in today's society comes from the Mass Media that has little regard for truth, Aquinas' approach appears to be both admirable and enviable.

Contraception is a barrier that separates the natural from the mysterious, thereby tending to enclose us within the natural. But the most memorable and dramatic moments, the most joyful moments of our life occur when the mysterious manifests itself through the natural. Contraception, therefore, is not liberating, but confining. It is never the subject of hymns, odes, celebrations, or festivities. It springs merely from a human choice, one that has no concern about converging with God's choice.

The word "procreation" relates to human creation that proceeds from God's creative Plan. The word "reproduction", on the other hand, implies that children are products of their parents who are the producers. As procreated, children are created in the image of God; as reproduced, they are produced in the image of their parents.

Contraception is part of a philosophy that implies that when it comes to having children, the husband and wife (or the producers) should be the only ones in charge. Psychologically, contraception conveys the attitude that if God is not in the picture when contraception is used, neither is He in the picture when intercourse is used without contraception.

Reproduction, rather than *procreation*, properly speaking, is not interested in God's Plan. Consequently, when contraception is put aside and a child is conceived, that child is regarded not so much as a child of God, but one of choice. At the same time, that child, in accepting his status as merely a child of his parent's choice, may sense, in some perhaps subtle way, that he is orphaned.

God's Plan embraces a convergence of choices, both the human and the Divine. Therefore, it incorporates both the natural and the mysterious. Conversely, from the human perspective, it includes intelligence and imagination, as well as faith.

Contraception is an attempt to disenfranchise God from the matter of creating new life and putting the responsibility solely in the hands of humans. But God remains the Author of life, and the contraceptive program, by disrespecting God's Plan, will deprive all its participants of blessings that they cannot afford to be without, and need far more than they realize.

Endnotes

[1] Thomas Aquinas, *Commentary of Pseudo-Dionysius on the Divine Names*, 4, 4.

[2] John F. Kippley, "Natural Family Planning: Questions and Answers," *Catholic Dossier*, Vol. 3, No. 5, Sept.-Oct. 1997, p.45.

[3] Kim A. Hardey, M.D., "Observations on My Life's Work," *op.cit.*, p.40.

[4] Germain Grisez, *The Way of the Lord Jesus: Vol.3, Difficult Moral Questions* (Quincy, IL: Franciscan Press, 1997), p.329.

[5] Viktor Frankl, *Psychiatry and Existentialism: Selected Papers on Logotherapy* (New York, NY: Simon & Schuster, 1967), p.21.

Contraception and Health

If married couples are offered the choice between practicing Natural Family Planning or Unnatural Family Planning, there can be little doubt that choosing the former would be the reasonable and realistic choice. But society does not always encourage people to make reasonable and realistic choices. This is especially the case when it comes to fertility regulation. Plato's Cave is still very much with us. We spend a great deal of time listening to "voices of authority" who, like the witches in *Macbeth*, are adept at making fair seem foul and foul seem fair. Natural Family Planning, then, is often cast in a negative light, as when it is disparaged as "Vatican Roulette." Unnatural Family Planning, on the other hand, is commonly eulogized as a breakthrough for "reproductive freedom."

Countering rhetoric with sound ideas can be very frustrating. Ideas are so casually dismissed, so frequently distrusted, and so easily misunderstood. It is often exceedingly difficult to disabuse the mind of long-held and firmly rooted errors, even if one is countering such errors with common sense. Pain, however, is a far more convincing experience. Teachers may feel helpless against the power of the reigning ideologies to impose illusions and obscure reality. But those who populate the doctor's waiting room or occupy hospital beds do not doubt the reality of their own pain. The trail of serious health problems that contraception has brought about constitutes a powerful and decisive argument that contraception is unnatural and therefore an unreasonable and unrealistic choice.

Promoting the Pill

Medical doctors who promoted the Pill in the early 1960's did so on the alleged basis that the Pill worked in harmony with nature. Their case had some degree of plausibility since it was developed from two female hormones: progesterone and estrogen. The Pill was therefore said to mimic the woman's natural monthly cycle. Synthetic hormones, however, are not the same as those that are produced naturally in the woman's body, and they have been demonstrated to have a decidedly different effect on female health.

The doctors who promoted the Pill were *not* unaware of the unnaturalness of putting synthetic hormones into a woman's body. They knew that the Pill worked by inhibiting the natural interaction of sex hormones and the pituitary gland. They were aware that since these interactions are so basic to life and health, the Pill was bound to produce significant deleterious effects. Moreover, scientists had established a connection between the sex hormone estrogen and cancer as far back as 1896. By 1932, it was known that estrogens and progesterone could cause changes in the breast, womb, ovaries, and pituitary glands in experimental animals.

By 1938, when Charles Dodds synthesized diethystilbestrol (DES) — the first inexpensive estrogen product that was potent enough to be taken orally — hundreds of studies of the carcinogenic features of estrogen had already been published (DES has been shown to cause breast cancer and vaginal cancer in the daughters of women who used it during pregnancy). The problem was not ignorance as much as knowledge being eclipsed by an inordinate eagerness to produce and promote a contraceptive in easy-to-take pill form that would prevent unwanted pregnancies (DES was not actually used to prevent pregnancy, but, mistakenly, to prevent miscarriage), safely, and effectively.

Doctors John Rock and Gregory Pincus, who developed the anovulent Pill in the 1950's, knew about the link between estrogen and cancer. They hoped, therefore, to produce an effective Pill that contained only the steroid progestin (its natural counterpart is called *progesterone*). Their all-progestin compounds, however, proved insufficiently effective. Women complained of episodes of excessive bleeding. In response, and with some regret, they then added estrogen to the Pill.

The "Combination Pill", as it was called, containing progestin and estrogen, was tested in Puerto Rico. One hundred thirty two women were involved. Three died from thrombosis, and many dropped out of testing. Very few of them received follow-up attention. The over-riding concern in this test, however, was not the health of the Puerto Rican women but the effectiveness of preventing unwanted pregnancies.

Given the disturbing side-effects associated with these "high-dose" Pills, such as blood clotting, disorders resulting in heart attacks and strokes, a "low-dose" Pill was produced that contained smaller amounts of estrogen. This new Pill reduced the frequency of these side-effects, although it brought about a greater incidence of ovulation, and consequently, of conception. More importantly, however, it introduced a new problem. Inasmuch as it did not always suppress ovulation, and because it rendered the endometrium lining of the uterus inhospitable for the implantation of the embryo, it often acted as an abortifacient. For many people who merely wanted a Pill that would prevent an unwanted birth, the distinction between a chemical contraceptive and a chemical abortifacient was not important. They did not object to the fact that they were practicing "abortifacient roulette." This attitude of indifference concerning whether one prevents or aborts a conception laid the ground for the social acceptance, later, of chemicals that were more specifically tailored to effect an abortion of the young embryo. RU-486, or the "morning-after" Pill, is a prime example of a chemical that does not prevent conception but aborts the conception that has already taken place.

The Side-Effects

The first major study of the general adverse effects of the Pill in the United States was done by Norman Ryder of the University of Wisconsin and Charles Westhoff of Princeton University. These two researchers, both sociologists, conducted their study for the United States Public Health Service.[1] They reported 1,603,500 episodes of disease among 8.5 million women who were on the Pill. Their reporting, nonetheless, did not include many of the more than fifty Pill-related diseases that the medical profession had documented by that time. Public health physician Dr. Herbert Ratner, who had a thorough knowledge of the literature, reported that a more realistic figure for the incidence of disease exceeded 10,000,000.[2] He pointed out that the incidence of thromboembolic deaths alone (from blood clotting) associated with the Pill was equivalent to the incidence of deaths in white women of childbearing age from crimes of violence which included murder, forcible rape, robbery, and aggravated assault.[3] The Federal Drug Administration (FDA) reported 227 Pill-caused deaths for the year 1969. Among the other diseases linked with the Pill are: thrombotic and hemorrhagic strokes, pulmonary embolism, depression, libido loss, vaginitis, chemical diabetes, and sterility.

It was becoming increasingly unconscionable for the scientific community to maintain that synthetic steroids acted in a natural way. Three doctors, from Harvard, Washington, and Columbia Universities, made the following rather forceful statement in their Preface to *Metabolic Effects of Gonadal Hormones and Contraceptive Steroids*: "Thus, in view of the qualitative and quantitative differences between the natural and synthetic steroids, we believe that semantic oversimplification which equates the pharmacological state induced by contraceptive steroids with biological states such as pregnancy should be abandoned."[4]

A *Newsweek* Gallup poll, February 9, 1970, reported that a startling two-thirds of Pill-taking women had not been informed by their physicians about the Pill's possible side-effects. It was on the basis of this apparent failure to respect a woman's right to be informed about the hazards of a powerful drug, that the Gaylord Nelson hearing on the Pill convened in Washington, D. C. in 1970. As a result of the Nelson hearings, the United States government required patient package inserts (PPI's for contraceptive Pills).

Two things had become clear: 1) the Pill was not safe; 2) women were not duly informed about the Pill's side-effects. Who was to blame? According to Harold Williams, M.D., LL.B., nearly everyone who was in a position of responsibility. In his monograph, *Pregnant or Dead? The Pill in New Perspective*, he declared that "The lay press, the medical press, medical organizations, drug companies, birth control enthusiasts, generally, and the Food and Drug Administration all must share the blame for the delays in revealing the facts about The Pill's sorry score on safety."

The government's requirement that PPI's be included with the Pill established an historical precedent and drastically altered the relationships between the drug industry, the FDA, the medical profession, and the consumer. For the first time, the government acknowledged that patients (female Pill users) were not expected to rely on their physicians for adequate information about the risks (or benefits) of a drug. Instead, the government required drug companies to provide this information directly to the patient.

Plato makes the distinction in his *Laws* between the physician who tends to slaves and the one who cares for freemen. The slave doctor prescribes his therapy "with an air of finished knowledge, in the brusque fashion of a dictator." The doctor of freemen, on the other hand, "treats their diseases by going into things thoroughly from the beginning in a scientific way, and takes the patient and his family into his confidence." Furthermore, he does not offer his prescription until he has earned his patient's support.[5]

The way that a doctor treats his patient indicates what he thinks of that patient and his right to be adequately informed. By withholding pertinent information and acting like a tyrant, the doctor expresses disdain for the patient as a free person and shows contempt for his right to be informed. Behaving in such a manner is tantamount to treating the patient as if he were a slave. Needless to say, this is an act of gross injustice.

There is a bitter irony in the fact that many women disregard the Pill's threat to their health in the name of reproductive freedom. In far too many instance, their expression of freedom led to their being treated as if they were slaves. In being willing to subordinate health to freedom, they lost their privilege of being honored as free. Choosing contraception is not, as many have been mislead into thinking, the same as choosing reproductive freedom. Countless women have discovered, to their dismay, that they subordinated their health not to freedom but to the illusion of freedom and the reality of disease. In her booklet, aptly titled, *The Pill and Liberation Mythology*, Melinda Reist contends that "It is more accurate to say that the Pill is in control — not the woman. . . . In the end, the Pill has subordinated and possessed her." [6]

Choosing the Pill to postpone initiation of a family, for example, can lead, as it has in many cases, to sterility. Commenting on this most unfortunate occurrence, Dr. Ratner has remarked that "There is no greater and more ironic retribution nature exacts than to rob The Pill user of the gift of motherhood she gratuitously takes for granted."[7] In an article under the poignant title, "Forever Babyless", the author recalls that "As a young woman contraceptives were my ticket to freedom. . . . Years later, longing for a child, I could hear my diaphragm mocking me in the night."[8]

Ethics and Ideology

Barbara Seaman complained, in her landmark report, *The Doctors' Case Against the Pill*, that there is something fundamentally wrong with a medical model that deems pregnancy, menopause, and not being pregnant as all being diseases. The unavoidable conclusion one must draw from this model, she noted, is that "*being a woman is a disease.*"[9]

One cannot lay all of the blame at the feet of the medical profession, however. When healthy women ask doctors, in the interest of avoiding pregnancy, to supply them with hazardous drugs, their request carries the implication that not being pregnant is a medically treatable condition, that is to say, a *disease*. The feminist ideology of "reproductive freedom" through medical intervention, actually welcomes medical exploitation. Healthy women, whose only complaint is that they do not want to get pregnant, invite doctors to treat them as if they had a disease. The doctors respond by giving them an ia-trogenic or physician-induced disease. Women then object that they have been exploited. This is hardly the path of liberation.

Added to this tragic combination of an unrealistic ideology and unethical medical practice is the opportunism of the drug compa-nies, deceptive advertizing, and the hyperbolic rhetoric of zero-populationists. Realism and good medicine are thereby obscured by the strategies of self-interest played out by a variety of competing groups. And female health is the biggest loser.

Dr. Ellen Grant, an obstetrician-gynecologist, and endocrinolo-gist, argued vehemently, in her book, *The Bitter Pill: How Safe is the Perfect Contraceptive?*, that the two Pill hormones, progestin and es-trogen, "would always cause too much illness."[10] In a later book, *Sexual Chemistry*, published in 1994, and reflecting another decade of careful research, she states flatly that "The contraceptive pill was never meant to be natural. A girl or woman taking the pill has sud-denly been temporarily medically castrated."[11] While some women were still protesting the "tyranny of their biology" that made preg-nancy a possibility, Dr. Grant was urging women to "reject the tyr-anny of the pill and other prescribed steroid hormones."[12]

Medical studies in recent years have confirmed the early research on the Pill that documented its risks. An article in the *American Jour-nal of Obstetrics and Gynecology* concludes that the low-dose Pill used by American women was a "massive uncontrolled experiment."[13] Recent case-controlled studies confirm the increase of thromboem-bolisms among Pill-users: "Compared with women not using oral contraceptives, current users of any type of pill had four times the risk of venous thromboembolisms [a blood clot that forms in the veins of the legs and may travel to the lungs]."[14]

The largest meta-analysis of studies showing the possible link between oral contraceptives and breast cancer reviewed 54 studies in 25 countries, representing more than 50,000 women who have breast cancer. It reported an increase of that pathology for women who used oral contraceptives.[15] (A meta-analysis is a synthesis of all ma-jor studies done in a particular field.) In other meta-analyses, one found that women who took oral contraceptive pills have a 42% in-creased risk of contracting breast cancer.[16] Another, more refined study, showed that women under 45 who had taken oral contracep-tives for four years or more prior to their first term pregnancy have a 72% increased incidence of breast cancer.[17] The four largest studies on this topic indicate that women under the age of 45 who took oral contraceptives before their first term pregnancy or within five years of menarche, showed at least a 40% (but as high as 88%) increased risk of breast cancer.[18]

A case-control study in Los Angeles indicates that the use of oral contraceptives doubles a woman's risk of developing adenocarcinoma of the cervix, with long-term users having the greatest risk. A Quebec study indicates a 40% increased likelihood of Pill-users to contract a late-stage precursor to cervical cancer, and this risk doubles among women who use the Pill for six years or longer. The World Health Organization (WHO) suggests that using the Pill increases the chance of developing cervical carcinoma *in situ,* and that long-term users are about twice as likely to do so as never-users.[19] Finally, "Participants who had used oral contraceptives within six months of the onset of ulcerative colitis were twice as likely to have the disease as those who had never used the pill."[20]

The statistics concerning the negative side-effects of the Pill, in all its many varieties, are impressive, consistent, and distressing. But they are nonetheless *statistics,* and as such are abstract and impersonal. Many people can find refuge in the illusion that "this is something that happens to others, but will not happen to me."

Individual cases sometimes speak more persuasively because their personal nature makes them more accessible to personal emotions, more identifiable with real life. The following examples may seem more real because they are personalized. But they are no less real than the countless instances of real human experiences that tend to get depersonalized when they are absorbed into a maze of statistical abstractions.

Leena Vadera began to experience some unpleasant side-effects of the Pill, including migraine headaches, dizzy spells and visual problems. Her doctor did not take these symptoms too seriously, passing them off as the result of the stress she was experiencing in anticipation of her wedding. Three days later, Miss Vadera suffered a stroke that left her completely paralyzed and able to communicate only with her eyes. She has initiated a law suit against her doctor.[21]

Judy Mozersky is also suing her doctor for similar reasons. The pill he prescribed for her in 1990, when she was nineteen, brought on, according to her attorney, the stroke that has left her paralyzed. She can communicate only by using eye blinks and eye movements.[22]

In Lille, France, Lens Hospital was ordered to pay $100,000 in damages to the husband and children of a woman whose death was caused by the use of RU-486.[23]

Deception

The epidemic of diseases attributed to the Pill and various chemical abortifacients, together with its train of permanent disabilities, and deaths is well documented and widely known. Dr. Malcolm Potts, apparently unaware that oral contraceptives, at the very least, should be placed under careful medical supervision, thinks that they should be sold over-the-counter. "As America looks at comprehensive health care," he writes, it has an exciting opportunity to save money currently wasted on supervising oral contraceptive use."[24] His statement is all the more astonishing since earlier in that same year, a Gallup survey reported that 86% of American women do not believe that oral contraceptives are sufficiently safe to obtain without a doctor's prescription.[25] The over-the-counter dispensation of oral contraceptives would not save money. Rather, it would send the cost of treating side-effects skyrocketing, not to mention the increased costs involved in law suits.

Nonetheless, medical deception continues and countless people are systematically misled. In 1995, the United Kingdom's Family Planning Association and the Health Education Authority launched a massive £1,000,000 publicity campaign to promote the morning-after pill. Attempting to mask the fact that this pill is an abortifacient, the Family Planning Association stated that "It is not an abortifacient", but merely makes "the lining of the womb disorganized and chaotic and unsuitable for a fertilized egg." What the Association does not want to explain is that making implantation impossible for the embryo, effectively aborts it. Moreover, what is aborted is not merely a "fertilized egg" of some undetermined species of animal, but a human being.[26]

Time and again one finds in medical and promotional literature the expression "emergency contraception" used to describe the use of various abortifacients. In a letter of protest to *Lancet*, a pharmacologist pointed out what all informed members of the medical profession really know, namely, that "emergency contraception" is "interceptive" in its functioning and not contraceptive.[27] The widespread practice of subsuming abortion under "emergency contraception" shows how the borders between contraception and abortion have become nearly invisible. This deliberate attempt at deception reveals only too clearly that contraception and abortion manifest a common mentality against life.

In July 1993, the Associated Press reported that the defect rate for condoms dispensed in Arkansas state health clinics and schools was more than 10 times higher than that tolerated by the FDA. United States Surgeon General Joycelin Elders, however, decided to keep the defect rate a secret since, in her view, it would "serve a greater public health purpose" to insure that the public did not lose confidence in condoms.[28] This is just one of many instances in which someone decides that a blind commitment to an ideology is more prudent than an enlightened commitment to the real health needs of human beings.

The prevailing dissatisfaction with oral contraception has provided ample reason for many to seek alternative forms of contraception. But, to their disappointment, none of the alternatives, provide a reliable way of preventing an unwanted pregnancy without causing adverse side-effects.

Norplant is a series of six nonbiodegradable silastic rods that are surgically implanted under the skin in the upper portion of the arm. It is a protocol for delivering a synthetic progesterone called levonorgestrel at low levels and in a sustained fashion into the patient's system. Norplant suppresses ovulation in roughly half of the menstrual cycles, but also suppresses the cyclic development of the endometrium. Thus, it works as an abortifacient. Norplant probably causes more side-effects than the Pill, although it may be more effective as a mechanism for avoiding unwanted births, especially for those who find difficulty in adhering to taking pills on a regular basis. But Norplant has not passed the satisfaction test. In one class action suit, 50,000 American women have complained of experiencing harmful side-effects.[29] In another class action suit, more than 800 Alabaman women sued the makers and distributors of Norplant, claiming that "the defendants knew the Norplant contraceptive caused health problems more severe and more frequent than those of comparable birth control methods.[30]

IUDs (intra-uterine devices) are poor contraceptives and can cause severe harm. The Dalkon Shield, originally hailed as a breakthrough in contraception, was later blamed for the deaths of 18 women and thousands of hyterectomies, infections, and spontaneous abortions before it was taken off the market. At the time it was withdrawn, A. H. Robins, the manufacturer of the Dalkon Shield, was spending $15 million a month in legal fees. The company's reorganization, which received final court approval, included the creation of a $2.5 billion fund to pay almost 200,000 Dalkon Shield claims.[31] Most doctors will not insert an IUD in a woman who has never borne a child since her uterine tone is high and she will most likely expel it.[32]

Diaphragms and condoms are also highly unreliable methods of preventing conception. Among adolescent condom users, unplanned pregnancies range from 18-26%.[33] Spermicides are also ineffective contraceptives and are not without their own sequelae of unpleasant side-effects.

It must also be noted that contraceptives, in general, leave their users more susceptible to contracting sexually transmitted diseases. Synthetic hormones, being immunosuppressive, are a threat to the immune system and facilitate the transmission of the HIV virus and other STDs.[34] Spermicides provide no additional protection against HIV or other sexually transmitted diseases than when condoms are used alone.[35] Condoms themselves are a weak defense against the HIV virus. The false security that contraceptives are effective and safe encourages more people to engage in sexual adventures, thereby increasing the pool of candidates who are eligible for STD infection.

There remains today no safe method of contraception. All forms of contraception pose significant health hazards in one way or another. Because of this, it is becoming more and more the case that the two most pervasive forms of fertility regulation are and will continue to be either sterilization and abortion or Natural Family Planning. In other words, the choice will more unequivocally be between Unnatural Family Planning and Natural Family Planning.[36]

The notion that women's health should be subordinated to "reproductive freedom" gives rise, in the real world, to some rather bizarre consequences and comparisons. Scholar Michel Schooyans has remarked that, in certain instances, there is less concern about the "hormonal force-feeding of women" than there is about the health of animals.[37] A story carried in the May 29, 1997 issue of the *New York Times* demonstrates the ironic truth of his remark.

Traditionally, the elephant population in South Africa is limited by natives who hunt them down for food. Administrators of South Africa's Kruger National Park decided to employ a more humane method of limiting the number of elephants by injecting them with Norplant. The contraceptive achieved its aim in preventing elephant pregnancies, but produced some unexpected and distressing side-effects. The Norplant left the female elephants in permanent heat. Their abiding interest became sex. As a result, according to the report, "Families have broken down. Two baby elephants have strayed from home because their mothers were permanently distracted." Given these unhappy consequences, authorities did the sensible thing. They discontinued the contraceptive program after it had been in effect for six months. The medical profession might be well advised to show at least the same consideration for its female human contraceptors.

Dr. Siegfried Ernst has commented that "Contraception expresses a lack of desire to subordinate sexual impulses to the will and plan of God."[38] The current willingness to subordinate health to one's sexual energies seems to be an inevitable consequence of this disordination. Once sexual energies become an end in themselves, divorced from health, love, family, and God's Plan, chaos, both morally and physically, is the natural result.

Sr. Hanna Klaus, MD, who is the Executive Director of the Natural Planning Center of Washington, D.C., offers sound medical and moral advice when she makes the following statement: "When one is treating a disease, one balances the risk of treatment against the risk of the disease itself. But fertility is not a disease; hence I do not believe that any risk to health is justified in coming to terms with it. The solutions are behavioral, not chemical or mechanical. To think otherwise is to imply that men and women are all powerless to direct and control their urges."[39]

We show respect for human beings when we honor their potentiality for putting their lives in order, that is, in living morally. We show respect for their bodies when we refrain from treating a natural and healthy condition they are blessed with as if it were a disease. We show respect for their lives when we encourage them to honor themselves and try to live a good and healthy life.

Despite the FDA's uneven record in matters of serving health interests, the motto for its official magazine is one that all medical personnel can live by, and is worth reiterating, reflecting upon, and putting into practice: "We are careful to preserve that life which the Author of nature has given us, for it was no idle gift."[40]

Endnotes

[1] C. F. Westhoff and N. B. Ryder, "Duration of Use of Oral Contraceptives in the United States," *Public Health Report*, 83: 277-87, April 1968.

[2]Herbert Ratner, "The Nelson Hearings on Oral Contraception — Testimony," *Child & Family*, Vol. 9, No.4, 1970, p. 356.

[3]*Ibid.,* p. 357; *Statistical Bulletin,* Metropolitan Life Insurance Co., Feb. 1968, p. 5.

[4]H. A. Salhanick, M. D. *et. al.* (ed.), *Metabolic Effects of Gonadal Hormones and Contraceptive Steroids* (New York, NY: Plenum Press, 1969).

[5]Plato, *Laws,* IV, 720 c-d.

[6]Melinda Reist, *The Pill and Liberation Mythology* (Stafford, VA: American Life League, 1992), p. 6.

[7]Herbert Ratner, "The Medical Hazards of the Birth Control Pill," *Child & Family*, Vol. 7, 1968, p. 79.

[8]Anne Taylor Fleming, "Forever Babyless," *Glamour,* July 1994, pp. 160, 170.

[9]Barbara Seaman, *The Doctors' Case Against the Pill* (New York, NY: Doubleday, 1980), p. xi.

[10]Ellen Grant, MB, ChB, DObstRCOG, *The Bitter Pill: How Safe is the 'Perfect Contraceptive'?* (London, England: Hamish Hamilton Ltd., 1985).

[11]Ellen Grant, *Sexual Chemistry: Understanding Your Hormones, The Pill and HRT* (London, England: Reed Consumer Books Ltd., 1994), p. 37.

[12]*Ibid.,* p. 268.

[13]Joseph W. Goldzieher, M. D., "Are Low-Dose Oral Contraceptives Safer and Better?" *American Journal of Obstetrics and Gynecology,* Sept. 1994, pp. 587-90.

[14]"Third-Generation Pills May Elevate Risk of Venous Thromboembolism," *Family Planning Perspectives,* June 1996, pp. 131-32.

[15]"Breast Cancer and Hormonal Contraceptives: Collaborative Reanalysis of Individual Data on 53,297 Women With Breast Cancer and 100,239 Women Without Breast Cancer From 54 Epidemiological Studies," *The Lancet,* Vol. 347, June 22, 1996, pp. 1713-27.

[16]D. B. Thomas *et al.,* "Oral Contraceptives and Breast Cancer: Review of the Epidemiological Literature," *Contraception,* 1991; 43:597-642.

[17]I. Romieu, *et al.,* "Oral Contraceptives and Breast Cancer," *Cancer,* 1990; 66:2253-2263.

[18]P. A. Wingo, *et al.,* "Age-specific Differences in the Relationship between Oral Contraceptive Use and Breast Cancer," *Cancer* (supplement), 1993; 71:1506-17. A. Rosenberg *et al.,* "Case-control Study of Oral Contraceptive Use and Risk of Breast Cancer," *American Journal of Epidemiology,* 1996; 143:25-37. L. A. Brinton, *et al.,* "Oral Contraceptives and Breast Cancer Risk among Younger Women, *JNCI,* June 1995; 87:827-35. E. White *et al.,* "Breast Cancer among Young U. S. Women in Relation to Oral Contraceptive Use," *JNCI, 1994; 86:505-514.*

[19]"Oral Contraceptive Users May Be at Some Increased Risk of Cervical Carcinoma," *Family Planning Perspectives,* Vol. 27, No. 3, May 6, 1995, pp. 134-36.

[20]"Pill Users May Experience Elevated Risk of Crohn's Disease, Ulcerative Colitis," *Family Planning Perspectives,* Vol. 26, No. 6, Nov.-Dec. 1994, pp. 281-82.

[21]"Paralyzed Woman Sues Pill Advice Doctor," *PA News,* Oct. 21, 1996.

[22]"Stroke Victim Doggedly Blinks Trial Testimony," *Pro-Life E-News Canada,* April 4, 1997.

[23]"The Facts: A Trial Won Against RU-486, Abortion Center, press release from La Trêve De Dieu, April 29, 1997.

[24]J. W. Gell, M. D. and Malcolm Potts, M. D., "Sell Birth Control Pills Over-the-Counter?" *Washington Times,* July 10, 1994, p. B4.

[25]"Contraception Jitters," *Ob. Gyn. News,* Feb. 15, 1995, p. 3.

[26]"Campaign to Camouflage Abortions," *Human Concerns,* No. 42, Summer 1995, pp. 1-5.

[27]Rolf G. Rahwan, "Morning-After Birth Control — Letter," *The Lancet*, Vol. 346, July 27, 1995, pp. 251-52.

[28]Winnipeg Free Press, Jan. 19, 1994.

[29]"The Culture of Death: Update," *Catholic Insight*, Jan.-Feb, 1997, p. 18.

[30]"More than 800 Alabama women sue Norplant," *Pro-Life News Canada*, Feb. 7, 1997.

[31]AP wire service story, "Dalkon IUD 'unfortunate,' ex-company president says," Sept. 12, 1990.

[32]Hanna Klaus, M. D., "The Reality of Contraception," *Catholic Dossier*, Vol. 3, No. 5, Sept.-Oct., 1997, p. 43.

[33]W. R. Grady *et. al.*, "Contraceptive Failure in the United States: Revised Estimates from the 1982 National Survey of Family Growth," *Family Planning Perspectives*, Sept.-Oct. 1986, pp. 200-09.

[34]Ellen Grant, *op. cit.*, 1985, p. 266.

[35]"BRF-Spermicide Study," *Associated Press*, April 4, 1997.

[36]Cf. Mercedes Arzu Wilson, *Love and Family* (San Francisco, CA: Ignatius Press, 1996), Part IV: "Natural vs. Unnatural Family Planning."

[37]Michel Schooyans, transl. John H. Miller, C. S. C., *The Totalitarian Trend of Liberalism* (St. Louis, MO; Central Bureau, 1997), p. 50.

[38]Dr. Siegfried Ernst, *Man, The Greatest of Miracles*, transl. Sr. M. Nathe, O. S. B. and M. R. Joyce (Collegeville, MN: Liturgical Press, 1976), p. 121.

[39]Hanna Klaus, *op. cit.*, p. 43.

[40]The author of the motto is Harvey W. Wiley.

Contraception and the Divided Self

The 1973 motion picture *Blume in Love* is about a husband (played by George Segal) who is desperately trying to win back his wife's love. There is a scene in which Blume makes a sexual advance toward his wife and is infuriated when she informs him that she is not using contraception. In a state of enraged incomprehension, he screams at her, protesting that the only people these days who do not use contraception are "Catholics and rapists."

This scene, in a mainstream movie, which some critics have given a "four star" rating (it is one of Roger Ebert's very favorites) is a good example of how brazen Hollywood can be in its ridicule of Catholics. At the same time, however, Catholics have become so inured by this form of media humiliation that the only people who might have found Blume's remark offensive were the rapists themselves. Catholics, whose views on contraception are presumed to be a public laughing stock, are thought to be as obedient to their dogma as rapists are to their hormones. But the "joke" is not funny as much as it is revelatory of Hollywood's shameless subservience to the *Zeitgeist*. And it also reveals how little Hollywood knows about what is really going on.

In that same year, 1973, anthropologist Lionel Tiger (neither a Catholic nor a rapist) wrote an article in an attempt to bring to light the fact that the Pill was wreaking havoc in the emotional lives of many women, including actresses. "What perversity has stimulated crash programs on the behavioral effects of marijuana," he asks, "but none on contraceptive drugs?" His article, "The Emotional Effects of the Pill" includes an impressive array of testimonies from women who complained about how the Pill adversely affected their emotional equilibrium.

A thirty-year-old actress confesses: "Just talking about the Pill depresses me. It took a long time to connect my being so down with being on the Pill, ... Never again, never again, will I put myself through that." "I felt completely cut off from my body, and especially from my sexuality," lamented a twenty-six-year-old newspaper reporter. And a twenty-four-year-old magazine editor reported: "During the entire time I was on the Pill I was subject to really extreme emotional outbursts. I felt like my body and emotions were simply out of control. . . . When I went off the Pill it took me a long time to feel good again, to feel in control of myself. Now I do, and I'll never go back on the Pill again."

Hormones influence behavior. The hormones the Pill contains not only influence behavior but the manner in which males and females see themselves as sexual beings, as well as how they view each other. The Pill affects not only sexual identity but how the sexes see fit to relate to one another.

The Pill achieves a "pseudo-pregnancy" and is often accompanied by symptoms associated with real pregnancy: nausea, weight gain, and water retention. It can also give rise to behavioral changes, causing depression, a lessening of sexual desire, and a confused concern about personal appearance together with an increased tension but decreased zest for doing anything to ameliorate the situation. Males, who tend to be more sexually attracted to women who are not pregnant but appear to be impregnable, are understandably confused by the signals they are getting from women who put themselves in a state of pseudo-pregnancy but exhibit the ill-effects common to a real pregnancy.

Twenty-four years later, Lionel Tiger was expressing the same concerns of male and female self-identities and the interaction between the sexes. In a *U.S. News and World Report* piece (July 1, 1996), the renowned anthropologist and evolutionary biologist re-confirmed what he had observed better than two decades ago. He acknowledge that tension between the sexes has increased since the Pill became available and that males are indeed more confused today about what it means to be a male.

Self-Division

It is neither humane nor scientific to dismiss all criticism of contraception as emerging from a narrow Catholic perspective. Nor are Catholics the only religious group that has voiced complaints against contraception. Consider, for example, three recent books against contraception authored by Protestants and written specifically for Protestant audiences: *The Protest of a Protestant Minister Against the Pill* by Rev. Matthew Trewhella; *Chemical Abortion* by Pastors for Life; and *Does the Birth Control Pill Cause Abortions?* by Randy Alcorn.

Contraception, whether in the form of the Pill or any or the many other varieties, raises anthropological concerns. How does contraception affect how a person thinks of himself as a sexual being? Does contraception separate the biological from the spiritual so that contracepting men and women begin to think of themselves as divided beings?

Lionel Tiger's observations, and those of other anthropologists, indicate that there is such a division, and it has an adverse impact on self-esteem, sexual relationships, marriage, and child-rearing.

"Man is a synthesis," wrote the Danish philosopher Søren Kierkegaard. He is a unity of body and soul, the biological and the personal. His freedom lies in being all that he is, a unification of the physical and the spiritual. But the prevailing notion of freedom in the modern world, strangely enough, is not in accepting one's wholeness, but in dividing oneself so that one part is free from the other. Underlying this self-division is the fear that one part is the enemy of the other. The following statement by a longtime user of contraception, who subsequently became a natural family planning practitioner, offers a lucid example of this self-division and the fear that it presupposes: "I used to think of my fertility as being something like a green monster lurking in a dark closet, ready to strike with a pregnancy at any time. For years I felt hopeless against the 'monster' unless I was 'armed' with the most powerful contraceptives on the market. What a sad, pathetic view to have held for so many years!"[1]

Walker Percy, who is best known for his novels, is an astute philosopher of cultural history. He was intrigued by the sharp dualism that marks the mentality of the modern world. Descartes, the Father of Modern Philosophy, gave modern philosophy its identifying trade mark — a radical dualism that divides man into two unmixable parts, one mind, the other, matter. Few have described this dichotomy as vividly as Percy has: "For the world is broken, sundered, busted down the middle, self ripped from self and man pasted back together as mythical monster, half angel, half beast, but no man."[2]

Contraception, which separates baby-making from love-making, is a form of radical dualism that perfectly mirrors the dualism of our time. And to be in step with the times, in this regard, is to be at odds with one's self. By pitting conception against sex, a kind of warfare within the self takes place. This warfare escalates through sterilization to abortion. Thus, babies are not the flower of interpersonal love, but enemies. Ellen Peck is only too candid in her best-selling book, *The Baby Trap*: "I want to tell you about this trap, not because I see babies as the enemies of the human race, really, but because I see babies as the enemy of *you*."[3]

This bizarre and self-defeating internal warfare has an interesting precursor in the animal world. The *bulldog-ant*, indigenous to Australia, is one of the oddest creatures on the face of the earth. If one cuts this unusual animal in half, the severed parts begin to war against each other. The head seizes the tail with its teeth, and the tail relentlessly defends itself by stinging the head. The battle may last for half an hour, until the parts expire or are dragged away by other ants.

The bulldog-ant both exemplifies and symbolizes what can happen when parts of the same living being are no longer harmoniously related to each other in the context of organic wholeness. Initially, there is a profound alienation characterized by a loss of the sense that the parts belong to the same being; next, and arising from this alienation, is an antagonism which sets parts against each other as mortal enemies.

This war between two parts of the bulldog-ant also provides an image of utter futility: the tail wants to destroy the head so that it can live as a tail alone, while the head wants to destroy the tail so that it can function as a head. The tragic law enacted here is that by attempting to dominate, the part can only destroy. In a war of the parts there can be no winners. In this way, alienation and antagonism combine to produce annihilation.

Has the human species evolved beyond the self-alienating potentialities of animals such as the bulldog-ant? Evolution, we might say, has not been kind to this Australian insect. But it is man himself, not evolution, that is the architect of the curious self-division he inflicts upon himself. The wisdom of wholeness is a value that seems to elude most moderns. It appears to be a casualty in the quest for control over one's body.

Control Over One's Body

The prevailing assumption that our own body, even when it is healthy and properly functioning, can rise up against us, suggests that, like a wild beast, it needs to be controlled. We get a strong sense of this negative image of the procreative potential of the human body in the following statement which one frequently finds in reading through the feminist literature of liberation: "I just could not allow myself to feel so much at the mercy of my biology. I was damned if I was going to let my body dictate the rest of my life."

Control over one's body, mind in charge of matter, seems to be a plausible path to freedom. The contradiction it represents, however, lies in the fact that part of one's own being is first disparaged and then enslaved. In speaking of her need for contraception, Rosemary Ruether has written that "It was essential to our whole plan of life to have control over biological potential so that we could plan the time when a child might be born. . . . one could not make commitments to foundations and colleges, if it was never possible to predict when a child would be born; . . . when there was no free choice, you could not stand upright and face the future, but only creep along on your belly from month to month as a kind of unwitting slave of biological fecundity."[4]

Mrs. Ruether's language is very strong, and her vivid imagery, especially the reference to the "belly" conjures up images of sub-human animals. But she seems to be a victim not so much of her body, but as a result of trying to control her body. Our body anchors us in reality and provides us with our natural mode of being and relating to others. Cut off from our body, we fancy that we are thereby made angels of some kind who can control the operations of the body, planning how many children to have and exactly when to have them. To quote Walker Percy once again, "chronic angelism-bestialism . . .rives soul from body and sets it orbiting the great world as the spirit of abstraction."[5]

It is a tragic illusion to think that we can have and avoid off-spring through acts of choice. It is not *choice*, an act of the will, but *sexual intercourse*, that invokes new life. We cannot command our body to be or not be fruitful. Contraception provides a perfect example of how we cannot yoke our body by a technology and then demand that it do our biding. As millions of people know through their own incontrovertible experience, a contraceptive does not always prevent a conception, and intercourse aimed at conception does not always result in new life. We cannot control our body. We cannot prevent its inevitable downward spiral toward death. We cannot control the aging process, nor can we immunize ourselves against all diseases and disabilities. We cannot *control* our body because our body is an inseparable part of who we are.

Control is indeed an essential part of human freedom and human dignity. Enslavement and degradation contradict the nature of the human person. But control is better directed not against our bodies but toward maintaining wholeness and ordering our lives so that they are in harmony with God's Plan and our own destiny. When we try to control our biology (and contraception is a good illustration of this), we turn against our selves. But when we try to control our actions in the interest of respecting and maintaining our wholeness as human beings, we are acting consistently and unambiguously for our own good. We may not succeed in getting what we want, but we can succeed in not dividing ourselves into two mutually antagonistic parts.

Simone de Beauvoir is the intellectual matriarch of contemporary feminism. Camille Paglia has said of her that her *magnus opus*, "*The Second Sex* remains for me the supreme work of modern feminism."[6] At Beauvoir's funeral, Elisabeth Badinter, her heir apparent, issued a cry that was repeated by many: "Women, you owe everything to her!"[7] Beauvoir's philosophy, which she derived almost holus-bolus from her friend and mentor, Jean-Paul Sartre, is an uncompromising glorification of liberty. But, as she writes, "There is one feminine function that is actually impossible to perform in complete liberty. It is maternity . . ."[8]

No one is a more ferocious critic of maternity than Simone de Beauvoir. What may be more intriguing, however, is not her contempt for marriage and childbearing, but her idealization of the career world. Like Sartre, and Descartes before him, she identifies the human with that purified, liberated abstraction that has rid itself of or separated itself from the enslaving power of matter. But such an abstraction, "no man", as Walker Percy says, is an illusion and not an existential subject that can enjoy anything, let alone "liberty." By denigrating her own body, she denigrates herself, creating an inner conflict that prevents (or even "contracepts", we might say), the flowering of true liberty. As C. S. Lewis has remarked, "We castrate and bid the geldings be fruitful."[9]

Our liberty, precious and desirable as it is, is conditioned by our reality. We are embodied creatures. This is our reality. We cannot achieve freedom if we reject our truth. It is our truth, then, that is the basis for our freedom. We become free *through* our body, not when we are separated *from* it.

Psychologist Judith Bardwick, in contrast with Beauvoir, understands that a woman's healthy sense of self requires that she accept the full reality of who she is: "The self-concept and self-esteem of women are closely linked to the appearance and function of their bodies because the life goals of women are closely tied to their bodies . . .Normal femininity includes the acceptance of menstruation, pregnancy, and maternity as the normal and desired consequences of being a woman."[10]

It is important, needless to say, to control our urges and impulses. But control does not imply a devaluation of that which is controlled. In the case of moral self-control, it implies integration. We control our urges and impulses not because they are inferior, but so that they can function properly within the context of our human wholeness. The moral purpose of control is not conquest but sublimation.

The career world is hardly a bed of roses or a fount of liberty. It is, quite often, a world of intense rivalry, venomous back-stabbing, and endless grievances. Its stresses, pressures, and tensions are so unremitting that survivors of the work week thank God it is Friday (TGIF). It is a world that literally cries out for a more peaceful and humane environment. Is it not the family, as Christopher Lasch has pointed out, that offers the only real haven in an otherwise heartless world?

Ms. Beauvoir is full of caution and advice for every potential mother since "an unwanted child can ruin her professional life."[11] Does she not know that the professional world can ruin her life, as well as that of her family? Does she see no dangers in the illusions that pride feasts on in a world that prefers abstractions to children?

The Path to Wholeness

The notion of a unified being does not mean very much to most people. It seems far too abstract, even though it does represent the fullness of a person's reality. Looking good and experiencing sexual pleasure for them *seem* to be more real. This attitude is evinced through interviews with people who continue to use contraception even when they experience its side-effects and are fully cognizant of its more serious risks.

"I know the Pill is dangerous," states one woman who took the Pill because she did not want to be flat-chested, "but I plan to stay on it come hell or high water." A medical librarian testified that she tried six different oral contraceptives over a three-year period, despite constant headaches, nausea, and leg cramps that used to wake her four or five times a night, because of what it did for her complexion. "My complexion had never looked so beautiful," she said. "All the little pores disappeared. I hardly needed makeup. A twenty-one-year-old woman protested: "I am not willing to give up sex, and I'm not willing to take the risk of getting pregnant." Another woman, well aware of the risks of the Pill, compared her attitude to the F. Scott Fitzgerald philosophy of "Live fast, die young, and have a good corpse."[12]

Mary Rosera Joyce has pointed out in *The Meaning of Contraception*, that "Contraception is not a matter of sacrificing the unity of one's being for the sake of love; it is a matter of denying this unity of being."[13] It is the person who loves, certainly not the person's parts. The sex organs in themselves are incapable of love. The more whole a person is, the better able he is to love. Marriage is at its best when it is between two people who not only value their wholeness — the unity of their respective beings — but offer them to each other as gifts. Contraception strikes against the wholeness of one's being and results in an impaired unity and a less than perfect gift.

Unity or wholeness is not something that people feel. It is, rather, who a person is. Feelings can create a momentary sense of strong unity, even when that unity has been compromised in its reality. We are often more sensitive to the lack of wholeness or authenticity we find in others than we are in noticing it in ourselves. Everyone prizes wholeness, but few practice it. Holiness itself is nothing more than a person living out the wholeness of his being.

To appreciate the value of one's wholeness requires a certain amount of wisdom. Philosophers, history's inveterate seekers of wisdom, have explained time and again that pleasure is associated with the part, but in order to be happy, to be filled with joy, one must be whole. The path to wholeness is ingeniously symbolized by the "Yellow Brick Road." In L. Frank Baum's perennially endearing story of *The Wizard of Oz*, the scarecrow, tin man, and lion each have enough wisdom to be acutely aware of the parts they lack: the scarecrow needs a brain, the tin man a heart, the lion courage. Even more to their credit, they ardently seek what they need in order to be more whole.

There can be little doubt that one reason for the broad and continuing appeal that *The Wizard of Oz* enjoys lies in the fact that Dorothy's curious companions characterize the very needs that plague modern society. We need a *brain* so that we can know what we need to know in order to direct our lives properly. Realistic ideas are crucial. They are, one philosopher remarks, "what enables man to live a life which is something above meaningless tragedy or inward disgrace. At the same time, it is only too common for people to submerge their capacities for realistic ideas, illuminating knowledge, and clear thinking under a torrent of emotionalism. If it "feels good, do it" better represents the contemporary ethos than "use your brain."

We need a *heart* so that we can love, so that we can extend to everyone the warmth of personal affirmation. Knowledge furnishes light, but love provides joy. Yet there is much discrimination, violence, and abuse in our society, and even marriage and the family, supposedly havens in a heartless world, are under attack.

We need *courage* so that we can face dangers, difficulties, and oppositions, without abandoning our commitment to what is right. Courage gives us the strength to stand by what we know and those we love. Nonetheless, the lack of courage in society is only too apparent. Alexander Solzhenitsyn has stated that the "decline in courage may be the most striking feature which an outside observer notices in the West in our days."[15] "Such a decline in courage," Solzhenitsyn went on to say, "is particularly noticeable among the ruling groups and the intellectual elite, causing an impression of loss of courage by the entire society."

We must view the scarecrow, tin man, and lion not as individuals who each seek one thing, but as a triumvirate or collectivity that seeks to integrate knowledge, love, and courage. In this regard, Plato was an ancient forefather. In his *Republic*, Plato spoke of man's "tripartite soul" which consists of *reason*, the reflecting principle, and *desire*, the unreflecting appetite, being coordinated through *spirit* which transmits the verdict of reason to desire and established a powerful bond between them.[16] In a similar way, C. S. Lewis states that "the head rules the belly through the chest."[17] The head alone is too abstract, cerebral. The belly alone is too animalistic, visceral, "The dream of many people, writes Erich Fromm, "seems to be to combine the emotions of a primate with a computerlike brain." But it is through the intermediary of the chest, or spirit, or courage, that man becomes fully a man.

The turbulent drama of sexual passion is not going to be brought under control by the mere dictates of reason. It requires something no less passionate than itself, a vibrant, animated courage, if it is to be integrated within the whole person. Knowledge and love will not be harmonized with each other in the absence of such a courage.

History makes it only too plain that the path to personal wholeness is indeed a long and crooked one. When ancient Egyptian embalmers prepared the Pharaoh's bodies for their journey to the next world, they performed their task diligently and lovingly. They believed that every organ had a special purpose and consequently preserved each one in a special way. There was one part of the body, however, for which they could not find any particular function. This was the brain, which the embalmers simply discarded. In the twentieth century, Albert Einstein willed that when he died, all of his remains be cremated *except* his brain. His disembodied brain is now housed in a research center in the Pyradomes, just north of Wichita, Kansas. After the passing of millennia, from the Pyramids to the Pyradomes, humanity is still merely a novice in the art of personal wholeness.

Particularly demanding of wholeness is the domain of human sexuality. Knowledge is needed not only in the personal sense to enable the spouses to become closer to each other, but also in the scientific sense to deepen one's awareness of reproductive physiology. Love is needed to fulfill and make fruitful the spousal relationship. Courage is needed to possess the strength to follow the path of knowledge and love, however unpopular or "politically incorrect" it may be in the eyes of the world.

The very expression, Natural Family Planning, may be seen as an integration of Knowledge, Love, and Courage. The Natural is an object of our Knowledge, the Family is formed in Love, and fidelity to the Planning requires no end of Courage.

Harmony of the parts characterizes Natural Family Planning, a harmony that commences with personal wholeness and progresses through marital intimacy and family unity as it moves toward communal solidarity. NFP, then, is evolutionary because it encourages its practitioners to attain higher forms of integration, while remaining faithful to their identities as persons.

A divided self is less than whole. Therefore, he is less happy and is less able to give everything he is. Contraception, in separating baby-making from love-making, is divisive of the self. But it also diminishes what the marriage partners are able to bring to each other. Contraception is neither a boon to the self or to marriage.

Endnotes

[1] Quoted in Nona Aguilar, *The New No-Pill No-Risk Birth Control* (New York, NY: Rawson Associates, 1986), p. 3.

[2] Walker Percy, *Love in the Ruins* (New York, NY: Dell Publishing Co., 1972), p. 360.

[3] Ellen Peck, *The Baby Trap* (New York, NY: Bernard Geis Associates, 1971), p.

[4] Rosemary Ruether, "A Question of Dignity," *What Modern Catholics Think About Birth Control*, William Birmingham (ed.), (New York, NY: The New American Library, 1964), pp. 234-35.

[5] Percy, *ibid.*.

[6] Camille Paglia, *Sex, Art, and American Culture* (New York, NY: Vintage Books, 1992), p. 112.

[7]Deirdre Blair, *Simone de Beauvoir: A Biography* (Simon & Schuster, 1990), p. 617.

[8]Simone de Beauvoir, *The Second Sex*, trans. H. M. Parshley (New York, NY: Alfred A. Knopf, Inc., 1980), p. 655.

[9]C. S. Lewis, *The Abolition of Man* (New York, NY: Macmillan, 1965), p. 35.

[10]Judith M Bardwick, *Psychology of Women: A Study of Bio-Cultural Conflicts* (New York, NY: Harper & Row, 1971), p. 73.

[11]Beauvoir, *op. cit.*

[12]Barbara Seaman, *op. cit., passim.*

[13]Mary Rosera Joyce, *The Meaning of Contraception* (Collegeville, MN: The Liturgical Press, 1969), p. 123.

[14]José Ortega y Gasset, *Mission of the University* (New York, NY: W. W. Norton, 1966), p. 37.

[15]Alexander Solzhenitsyn, *A World Apart; an address given at the Harvard Commencement Exercises*, June 8, 1978 (St. Paul, MN: Wanderer Press, 1978), p. 4.

[16]Plato, *Republic*, IV, 435-42.

[17]C. S. Lewis, op. cit., p. 34.

Contraception and Compromised Intimacy

In *Beyond God the Father*, feminist author Mary Daly argues that original sin was a good since it represented a "Fall into Freedom."[1] Her remark reflects three positions of fundamental importance that are now deeply imbedded in the collective psyche of contemporary society: 1) the denigration of fatherhood; 2) the absolutization of freedom; 3) the rejection of marriage as a permanent and uncompromised form of intimacy between husband and wife. Contraception is congenial to each of these positions. It prevents fatherhood from coming to be, it protects the freedom of the individual from the responsibilities of parenthood, and it separates husband and wife from each other so that their degree of intimacy with each other is at least compromised.

In *Crossing the Threshold of Hope*, John Paul II states that original sin is a fundamental evil which, in attempting to abolish fatherhood, establishes a direction that can lead only to a "master-slave relationship."[2] For the Holy Father, contraception compromises intimacy between man and God, and between husband and wife. Moreover, this compromise leads away from freedom.

Does contraception lead toward or away from freedom? This question cannot be answered realistically apart from understanding the relationship that exists between freedom and love. If freedom simply means separation from others or pure individuality, then love would actually hinder such a form of freedom. But without love, man is in a state of misery. Therefore, the freedom he seeks cannot exist without love. Love guides and directs freedom to what is good. To love another person means to use one's freedom in the interest of securing the other person's good. In this sense, freedom is not a terminal value but something that allows a good to be realized.

Contraception compromises the intimacy between husband and wife because it negates part of their being, in particular, that which is ordered to procreation. Another way of expressing this "compromise" is to say that the unselfishness of their spousal love is diluted by the presence of self-interest. The dominant philosophy of the secular world, however, does not regard such self-interest as problematic. As a spokesperson for this philosophy, Elizabeth Badinter, in her book, *The Unopposite Sex: the End of the Gender Battle*, states that "the categorical imperative no longer sets out the conditions of the relationship between Ego and Other People, but those of my relationship with myself. It orders me to love myself, to develop myself, to enjoy myself." For Badinter, the moral code has shifted from the Other to Oneself, making the Ego absolute and rendering relationships valid only insofar as they serve the Ego.

Contraception is consistent with this withdrawal into the self, as well as a withdrawal from God the Creator of Life. Pope Paul VI fully recognized this shift toward the Ego and was profoundly saddened by the radical under-appreciation of love it presupposed: "In love there is infinitely more than love. We would say that in human love there is divine love. And that is why the link between love and fecundity is deep, hidden, and substantial! All authentic love between a man and a woman, when it is not egoistic love, tends toward creation of another being issuing from that love. To love can mean 'to love oneself,' and often love is no more than a juxtaposition of two solitudes. But when one has passed beyond that stage of egoism, when one has truly understood that love is shared joy, a mutual gift, then one comes to what is *truly* love."[3]

"Juxtaposition of two solitudes" is a most poignant expression. It succinctly captures the frustration of performing an act which is designed to bring about unity while retaining sufficient self-interest to fall back on one's isolated self. This contradiction has been duly noted by a number of distinguished artists.

Alienated Lovers

The contemporary surrealist painter René Magritte, whose work offers some of the most disturbing images of alienation and fear in the lexicon of modern art, captures the contradiction of non-intimate intimacy in his painting *The Lovers*. Here Magritte portrays a man and a woman posing to kiss each other; but their amorous endeavor is an icon of frustration since their heads are wrapped in gray cloth integuments. They are 'lovers', and yet remain anonymous and alienated.

C. S. Lewis, in *That Hideous Strength*, describes a form of love-making among a particular tribe of people that represents the logical extreme of marital alienation: "When a man takes a maiden in marriage, they do not lie together, but lie with a cunningly fashioned image of the other, made to move and to be warm by devilish arts, for the real flesh will not please them, they are so dainty (*delicati*) in their dreams of lust."[4]

Walker Percy carries this theme of alienated love-making even further by completely dissociating the 'lover' from a human partner. In one scene in his novel *Love in the Ruins*, a woman goes to the "love clinic" where, attached by Lucite fittings to sensor wires, she is connected to her 'lover' which is a computer.[5]

Eugene Ionesco has a scene in his play, *The Bald Soprano*, in which a man and a woman meet by chance and proceed to engage in a most revealing conversation. They discover that they both took the ten o'clock train to New York from New Haven that morning, both have a seven-year-old daughter, both live in the same building on Fifth Avenue, and, both, in fact, live in the same apartment. They realize to their astonishment that they are married to each other. This realization is made not through mutual recognition, but by a process of logical deduction.

In Milan Kundera's novel, *The Unbearable Lightness of Being*, the protagonist tries to lead a sexually active life while remaining detached from any personal responsibility or commitment. His ideal is to free himself from all moral chains so that he can float from one conquest to another. By the end of the novel he discovers that his ideal has betrayed him. His "lightness of being", which is really a flight from his substantial self, has become truly unbearable.

The movie, *Paris, Texas*, centers on a man who is bent on finding his estranged wife. The man is played by Harry Dean Stanton, who has been described as the most forlorn and angry of all great American character actors. After a long and arduous search, he finds her. She is working in one of those sleazy emporia where men pay to ogle women and to speak to them on the telephone. The Stanton character finds himself seated only a few feet away from his wife. Emotionally, they are light-years apart. The one-way mirror that allows him to see her, but does not allow her to know who is viewing her, is a powerful symbol of contraception. It prevents even a visual intimacy. It shows marriage as a microcosm of alienation set within a society in which alienation seems to be accepted without question.

Contraception allows sexual partners to go through the motions of being intimate without their being truly intimate, that is, unreservedly and unconditionally so. The fact that contraception is perfectly in accord with the dominant tone of an alienated society means that the general populace scarcely notices its intrusion upon their intimacy, although it cannot help but notice the consequences of this intrusion in the trivialization of sex, the weakening of the marital bond, the increase in infidelity, the decline in the birth rate, and the sharp rise in the rate of women who conceive and abort unwanted offspring.

An intriguing example of how oblivious a person can be to the processes of alienation is brought to light in a letter to Abigail Van Buren, America's most popular advisor to the lovelorn. An unusual feature on this occasion is that although the letter was published, Dear Abby could not think of any way to respond to it.

> I am a twenty-three-year-old liberated woman who has been on the pill for two years. It's getting pretty expensive and I think my boyfriend should share half the cost, but I don't know him well enough to discuss money with him.[6]

The "liberated" woman is somehow more confident that she can communicate better with a stranger than she can with her live-in 'lover'. She is oblivious to her own inner alienation, how her verbal and sexual modes of communication are separated from each other. What appears to bother her most is not her own personal disorder, the illusion that she is "liberated", or that her most trusted confidante is a person who does not know her, but that she is paying too much for contraception.

Abby might have taken the time to explain to her anxious writer that a divided self is not a candidate for a unified relationship. Self-division has no potential for intimacy with another. But in stating this, she would no doubt anger many of her readers, especially those who would perceive the central issue is one of sexism rather than personal alienation.

Bonding vs. Bondage

Central to a philosophy of individualism is the notion that intimacy between two people compromises individuality. According to this view, the distinction between bonding and bondage is academic. Even the bond of matrimony is regarded as a form of bondage.

Contraception promises to liberate couples from the bondage of pregnancy so that they can better enjoy each other as persons. But a person is not a bodiless soul, nor is pregnancy necessarily a form a bondage.

The denigration of bonding because it is presumed to be incompatible with the freedom that is associated with liberation from the body is essentially anti-human. The body is an integral part of the human identity. It is primarily through the body that we are who we are and know others as they are. It is through the body that we meet others. Human beings do not function very well as disembodied egos. They suffer acutely from separation reactions. "No-relatedness", as psychiatrists aver, is both unnatural and unbearable. Contemporary novelists insistently and persistently call their readers' attention to the existential plight of modern man who is separated from community (isolation), from tradition (dislocation), from persons (alienation), from meaning (emptiness), and from hope (despair). Collectively these various separations create an illusion of freedom. This freedom, however, is a freedom from the very facts and forces that are the formula for his humanization. "You are not free unless you are bound," as the philosopher Karl Jaspers exclaims. A tree is obviously not free to be itself if it is unrooted from the soil, shielded from the sun, shorn of leaves, and deprived of all nourishment. To be a tree, it must be bound to what feeds and sustains it.

The modern dilemma unfolds when people are freed from every form of connectedness in the interest of achieving freedom only to find that the resulting dissolution leads straight to misery. Is it possible to achieve freedom and yet escape misery? Or, conversely, is it possible to avoid misery without falling into bondage? Are freedom and happiness compatible?

Philosophy is entirely useless if it does not make distinctions. Bonding is not the same thing as bondage. The latter is restricting and frustrating, contrary to one's natural needs. It is in no way compatible with true freedom. Bonding, on the other hand, if it is directed by love to a good, can be the beginning of an expanding freedom. Bonding is an adherence to that which overcomes our isolation and alienation and completes us. Friendship is a bond that we cannot do without.

Bondage and bonding do have something in common; they both involve connectedness. But bondage is stifling, connecting people with something that hinders them. Bonding can be liberating if it is interpersonal and protected by love. The philosopher Benedict Spinoza understood bondage to be the consequence of making desire absolute. It was this notion of bondage that inspired Somerset Maugham's novel about the enslaving potentials inherent in sexual lust — *Of Human Bondage*.

There is no disputing the fact that bondage exists. By contrast, bonding is far more subtle and mysterious, though the evidence for its existence is decisive. It is well known, for example, that animals bond with their young. To cite but one instance, experiments have shown that if a litter of rabbits is taken from the mother, she will exhibit a demonstrable shock response at the very moment individuals from the litter are killed. Moreover, this response is registered even when the victim rabbit is hundreds of miles from its mother.

Bonding between humans includes moral and spiritual dimensions that sometimes elude a strict materialistic analysis. Nonetheless, interpersonal bonding can be authenticated on a bio-chemical level where it appears in its most natural and spontaneous form. There are essentially three kinds of such bio-chemical bonding between humans: sexual intercourse, pregnancy, and lactation. Each of these is ordered to the next in such a way as to promote the development of both the child as well as the relationship between the parents. In this sense, bio-chemical bonding is consonant with an emerging freedom.

It is well established, scientifically, that both male and female derive physiological benefits to their health by the absorption of each other's secretion during sexual union. The assimilation of hormones which the female organs pass to the man's body through the permeable mucous membranes of the male organ, and the assimilation of the male semen and its hormones through the mucous membranes of the female organ play an important role in the satisfying functioning of other physical and emotional processes that contribute to a harmonious married life.

Dr. Marie Stopes recognized early in the twentieth century that a woman suffered a loss of well being when deprived of her husband's seminal and prostatic fluid. She reported her findings, which were later corroborated by other medical researchers, in 1919 in her book, *Wise Parenthood*. She opposed *coitus interruptus* and the use of the condom precisely because they deprived the sexual act of its full physiological value.

Contraception can be viewed, if not as a form of compromised intimacy between husband and wife, at least as an impediment to achieving a fuller two-in-one-flesh bonding. Sexual intercourse is ordered to ends other than procreation even on a physiological level. It confers a multitude of benefits on the partners that all contribute in their own way to facilitating the special bond of unity between husband and wife that is, in a very fundamental sense, the bond of matrimony.

Regrettably, sexual intercourse is often viewed solely in terms of the psychological benefits it confers upon the individual. A TV character illustrates the point perfectly when she says to her friend, "I do it for the 'endolphin' rush." Her friend gently corrects her: "You mean the *endorphin* rush!" According to today's social etiquette, it is permissible to correct a person for misusing a word, but not for misusing her body.

Apart from the evident relationship between intercourse and conception, intercourse has a crucial role to play in modifying a woman's immune system so that it does not regard semen as a foreign substance it must protect itself against. Male semen contains a mild immunosuppressant that instructs the woman's immune system to accept its ingredients as well as the child that may subsequently be conceived. In other words, the immunosuppressant carried in the semen signals the woman's body not to reject but to bond with her husband and the child to come. This is an indication that a special monogamous intimacy is taking place between husband and wife on as fundamental level of their being as their immune system. According to Dr. Alan Beer of the Chicago Medical School: "there is now strong evidence" that a father's semen contains a "molecular message" which may be necessary to "initiate the immune chain of events associated with the 'immunoprotection' of the baby."[7] The father's semen, therefore, prepares the woman's immune system to "recognize" the peculiar chemical composition of her husband's semen and the forthcoming child as somehow belonging to her and therefore exempt from being attacked as foreign objects.

Compromised Intimacy

Sexual union is a two-in-one-flesh intimacy that requires the complete surrender of the spouses to each other. Contraception compromises this intimacy. It is a way of holding back, of not giving everything one has and not being prepared to accept all the consequences that flow from an act of undiluted sexual union. Those who employ contraception usually do so in the interest of gaining some measure of control over their lives. But this desire for control is somewhat illusory since it usually means a willingness to give oneself to something other than the marriage itself. Spouses often compromise their marital intimacy so that they do not compromise their intimacy with something else. This other "intimacy" is frequently a certain standard of living.

Dr. John Schimel reports the following dream of one of his patients:

> I am in bed with my wife, and between us is my accountant. He is going to have intercourse with her. My feeling about this is odd — only that somehow it seemed appropriate.[8]

One must always be cautious, needless to say, when it comes to interpreting dreams. Dream analysis is far from an exact science. Nonetheless, this patient's dream provides a coherent symbol of how an excessive concern for material security can compromise a husband and wife's intimacy.

The accountant in the dream personifies financial concerns. The husband's acquiescence to his wife's intimacy with him suggests that the husband has given his approval to such an arrangement. The arrangement seems "odd" to the husband, probably because he does not want to admit it to himself on a conscious level, although he has pushed the matter into his subconscious. Contracepting couples may not recognize the subtle erosions that contraception brings about. Sometimes the reality is too unpleasant for them to admit on a conscious level.

In Paul Claudel's play, *Soulier de Satin* (*The Satin Slipper*), the heroine leaves her shoe behind in the bedroom where her marital infidelity takes place. The symbolic meaning for the playwright here is to indicate that the woman will be maimed by her indiscretion, and from that moment on will always walk with a limp. Infidelity must leave a scar.

The motion picture *Indecent Proposal* shows, in rather convincing fashion, how an inordinate desire for money can have a destructive impact on a marriage. In the film, the married couple (played by Demi Moore and Woody Harrelson) agree that the wife's one-night stand with a wealthy tycoon (played by Robert Redford) in exchange for a million dollars, is an intelligent choice. The young married couple believes that the money gained by the transaction is a far greater good than any minor problem that might arise from a single act of wifely infidelity. What the husband and wife soon discovered, through excruciating pain, was that marital intimacy is uncompromisable in its nature. They discovered that once they allowed inroads into their intimacy, even for a seemingly cogent reason such as the acquisition of a million dollars, their entire marital framework quickly began to disintegrate. Their greed betrayed them. It was as if they thought they could wound a thoroughbred horse in the leg and still expect him to run a strong race. Marital intimacy must remain inviolate if it to function properly.

Subordinating the unity of one's marriage to a monetary interest, even for one night, means that one's primary commitment is to money and not to one's marriage, a preference for the impersonal over the personal. The recognition of this moral inversion precipitates feelings of shame, anger, and betrayal. Compromised intimacy, whether through sexual infidelity or through an excessive concern for something alien to one's marriage, can bring about an identity crisis. Who am I? Am I a husband, a wife, an opportunist, a social climber, a traitor?

Sean Connery and Diane Cilento, as explained on television's *David Susskind Show*, decided to marry each other primarily to save money on air travel, since, at that time, a wife was entitled to accompany her husband for half-fare. It is only too clear that placing the basis of one's marriage in the hands of airline personnel who regulate the price of tickets, is to side-step the issue of intimacy altogether as well as to surrender control of the fate of one's marriage to an external and arbitrary agency. The continuation of the marriage thereby becomes highly unlikely. The airlines ultimately discontinued their policy of offering wives half-fare; the Connery couple discontinued it marriage.

The family is the basic unit of society. More fundamentally, marriage is the basis of the family. Even more fundamentally, a loving, intimate union of husband and wife is the basis of a good marriage. Therefore, the uncompromised intimacy between spouses establishes a solid foundation for society. A good marriage, as Professor William E. May asserts, is the "rock on which the family is built." "Children can flourish fully," he states, "only in the family rooted in the marriage of one man and woman. Only if this truth is recognized can a 'civilization of love' be developed."[9]

"Only our failures only marry," said M. Carey Thomas, the first dean and second president of Bryn Mawr College. This is Ms. Carey's sophisticated way of demeaning women who marry. Such chauvinistic feminism, however, is blind to the essential importance marriage and the family have for society. It also fails egregiously to recognize the creative as well as indispensable role that married couples are called to play.

Creative Intimacy

Contraception is contrary to the natural law, poses significant health risks, causes division within the self, inclines toward selfishness, and compromises marital intimacy. This seems to be a very high price to pay in order to prevent unwanted pregnancies. But contraception does not always succeed in this regard. One may pay this very high price, then, and not secure the one advantage that is supposed to offset all the disadvantages.

Natural Family Planning, on the other hand, is an effective and reliable means of regulating fertility, but without any of the physical side-effects or the demoralizing features associated with contraception. Natural Family Planning honors the integrity and intimacy of the married couple. Dr. Wanda Poltawska, of the Institute for the Theology of the Family in Krakow, Poland, uses Natural Family Planning as therapy for couples who have become alienated by contraceptive sexual intercourse.[10] Nona Aguilar reports in her book, *No-Pill No-Risk Birth Control*, of couples whose relationships improved once they abandoned contraception and adopted Natural Family Planning. As one woman who spoke for many said: "I now know the true meaning of the word 'intimate'."[11]

There are two basic desires that are innate in man: a desire for the infinite and a desire for the intimate. These desires are very powerful and often interfere with each other. The infinite without the intimate is abstract; the intimate without the infinite is unsatisfactory. Our appetite for the infinite is boundless; our appetite for the intimate is only too quickly quenched. The great problem in life is how to reconcile them. In pursuing the infinite without the intimate, one is likely to sacrifice a person for an abstract ideal. In Henrik Ibsen's *When We Dead Awaken*, Rubek sacrifices Irene for an artistic ideal. In Nathaniel Hawthorne's *The Birthmark*, Alymer sacrifices his wife, Georgiana for an aesthetic ideal. On the other hand, one may pursue the intimate to the exclusion of the infinite. In this regard, Don Juan tries desperately to find satisfaction in being intimate with a number of women. Calypso wants to possess Ulysses; Ulysses wants to possess the Sirens. Greed wants the infinite, but spurns the intimate. Lust is riveted to the intimate, but detests the infinite.

Through marital intimacy the desires for the intimate and the infinite are reconciled. One is intimate with his spouse while at the same time is in touch with God the Infinite Being who creates life through moments of human intimacy. Loving union between spouses, therefore, is creative not only inasmuch as it brings new human life into being, but also because, in reconciling the fundamental desires for the intimate and the infinite, it assists in the creation of whole human beings.

Sexual intimacy intimates the infinite. To affirm this order is to affirm the fundamental order of creation. To violate it, which contraception does, is to make the infinite inaccessible and to make an idol of the intimate.

The Old Testament uses the word *yadoah* (to know) for the act of sexual union. Knowledge and sexual love have an important factor in common in that they both imply an entering into something that exists outside the self. The knower is united with the object of his knowledge and his knowledge is objective to the degree it is free from subjective prejudices and biases. The true knower knows his beloved as he is and not as he might prefer him to be. Likewise, the true lover will love his partner as he is, without altering his being to suit some convenience or security need. In this same sense, the ancients proclaimed *"ubi amor, ibi oculus"* — where there is love, there is also vision (knowledge).

By taking knowing and loving together — *yadoah* — a special intimacy is achieved between husband and wife in which each knows and loves the other with reverence, that is, with respect for the way they are. This *yadoah* intimacy is the basis for creativity in the married life of husband and wife, in the life of the species, and in the continuing life of the community.

Intimacy requires knowledge and love in the strictest sense of these terms. But knowledge and love need courage, and courage needs faith. If there should be one sacrosanct, uncompromisable, inviolate relationship between people in all of society, it should be the sexual union between husband and wife. Marriage, then, demands extraordinary and well-developed virtues. Accordingly, one woman writer states that "marriage is the hallowed ground, the sanctified place for those lovers who should, who are able, who are permitted and who are determined to take the risk of procreation."[12] Marital intimacy is difficult and menaced on all sides. Yet its difficulties pale when compared with its rewards, for it is the antidote *par excellence* for loneliness, selfishness, fear, and alienation. And it is the ordinary and unsurpassable means of conceiving new life, and by virtue of that new life, offering a weary world new hope.

Society begins when a man and a woman promise one another love and fidelity, a promise that anticipates an abundance of communal benefits that is the shared offspring of their creative intimacy.

Endnotes

[1]Mary Daly, Beyond the Father: Toward a Philosophy of Women's Liberation (Boston, MA: Beacon Press, 1973).

[2]His Holiness John Paul II, Crossing the Threshold of Hope, ed. Vittorio Messori, trans. Jenny McPhee and Martha McPhee (New York, NY: Alfred A. Knopf), p. 228.

[3]*The Pope Speaks: Dialogues of Paul VI with Jean Guitton*, tr. by Anne and Christopher Fremantle (New York: Meredith Press, 1968), p. 275.

[4]C. S. Lewis, That Hideous Strength (London: Pan Books, 1961), pp.166-67.

[5]Walker Percy, Love in the Ruins (New York, NY: Dell, 1972), p. 118.

[6]Abigail Van Buren, The Best of Dear Abby (New York, NY: Andrews & McMeel, 1981), p. 242.

[7]Journal of the American Medical Association, Dec. 8, 1989.

[8]Dr. Schimel, as quoted in Rollo May, Love and Will (New York, NY: Norton, 1969), p. 38.

[9]William E. May, Marriage: The Rock on which the Family is Built (San Francisco, CA: Ignatius Press, 1995), p. 37.

[10]See Fr. Anthony Zimmerman, S. V. D., "Why Marriages Disintegrate When Contraception is Used," Fidelity, Feb. 1983.

[11]Nona Aguilar, No-Pill No-Risk Birth Control (New York, NY: Rawson & Wade, 1980), p. 102.

[12]Ida Friederike Görres, Zwischen den Zeiten (Olten: Walter, 1961), p. 64.

Contraception and
the Trivialization of Sex

The experience of fragmentation has shaped the artistic and moral sensibility of our epoch. World Wars I and II, and all the innumerable regional wars that followed have brought to modern consciousness a searing image of a world that has been shattered and ripped to pieces. Order has yielded to disorder, continuity has been replaced by dicontinuity, cosmos has given way to chaos. We now live in the *Atomic Age*, the *Age of Anxiety*, a *Post-Christian World* in which God is presumed to be dead. Families are uprooted, industrialized labor is piece-meal, ethics is anti-nomian. University educators routinely teach that meaning, religion, law, and morality have all been *deconstructed*.

In the words of the Irish poet, William Butler Yeats, "Things fall apart; the centre cannot hold; Mere anarchy is loosed upon the world." Prominent psychologists speak of our "collective death wish", while philosophers harp incessantly about the problem of alienation. And sociologists decry the rapidly diminishing number of face-to-face relationships there are within society. Pope John Paul II diagnoses the contemporary climate as a "culture of death."

If we were to seek a visual image that adequately epitomizes our fragmented world, we could not find a better one than Picasso's 1937 painting, *Guernica*. In this large mural, Picasso depicts, as symbolic of the depersonalizing fragmentation of the modern world, the devastating effect of Nazi *blitz-krieg* on this small Spanish town. What artist captures more vividly the de-composition of the twentieth century world? According to one critic: "In Picasso's pictures we feel the real pain of the world's coming apart, layer by layer, the world's dematerialization and decrystallization, the atomization of the world's flesh, the rending of all the veils."[1]

In 1941, four years after Guernica, Pope Pius XII addressed the judges of the Roman Rota on an important moral issue. He was deeply concerned about the effect a climate of fragmentation would have on attitudes toward human sexuality. In retrospect, one would have to agree that his words were remarkably prescient:

51

. . .there are two tendencies to be avoided: first the one which, in examining the constituent elements of the act of generation, considers only the primary end of marriage, as though the secondary end did not exist, or were not the *finis operis* established by the Creator of nature himself; and secondly, the one which gives the secondary end a place of equal principality, detaching it from its essential subordination to the primary end — a view which would lead by logical necessity to deplorable consequences.[2]

The Importance of Order

Pius XII feared the fragmentation, "layer by layer", of human sexuality. Therefore, he denounced the divorce between the unitive aspect of sexual intercourse that united husband and wife in a profoundly personal way from the procreative end that invoked God's creative Hand. He denounced procreation without personal love because it disparaged the physical and interpersonal dimensions of sexual union that God himself had created. He denounced sexual union that negated the possibility of procreation for a more complex reason. As he stated, he feared the "deplorable consequences" that would eventuate if the secondary end of marriage — the good of the act of intercourse for the spouses — was no longer "subordinated" to the primary end which is to honor the generative implications of the sexual act.

By subordinating the secondary end of sexual union to the primary end, Pius XII was merely restating a long and firmly-held tradition. The Code of Canon Law, in the famous Canon 1013, states: "The primary purpose of marriage is the procreation and education of children. The secondary purpose is mutual support and a remedy for concupiscence." He was not suggesting, nor did he hold, that one end is superior or more excellent than the other, but was simply indicating that the integrity of the marital act demands an ordination of one part to the other. To reject this order is to violate the integrity of the act. This notion of order, how one thing naturally leads to another, is what the modern world has great difficulty in comprehending. In an epoch of fragmentation, contraception, which separates the two ends of the marital act from each other, seems to unlock a door of freedom. How could "deplorable consequences" spring from an act of freedom?

St. Augustine defined peace as the "tranquility of order." Life itself is a series of orderly steps and stages. Putting one's life in order is a minimal condition for a meaningful life. "It belongs to the wise man to order," as St. Thomas remarks. Breaking up the natural order of things removes each element from its web of meaning. As order is disrupted, meaning becomes eroded. Marriage and sexual union between husband and wife are a matter of such incomparable importance that one must be extremely wary of what dire consequences or altered meanings might follow upon the disruption of its natural ordination.

In farming, the order of planting, cultivating, and harvesting is established by nature and cannot be altered. To say that planting is subordinated to harvesting is to say that the latter fulfills the purpose of the former. But it is also to say that harvesting gives meaning to planting. Can one separate the two ends of marital union without radically altering their meanings?

Preposterousness

The common usage meaning of the word "preposterous" refers to something that is contrary to nature, or absurd. Its etymology offers an important additional insight to this meaning. Derived from the Latin words, *prae* (before) and *posterius* (after), it literally means putting *before* that which comes *after*. Preposterousness, then, has to do with a change in order. It is, so to speak, putting the cart before the horse, or bolting the barn door after the animals have escaped.

Preposterousness in the moral domain has a particularly important ramification. When something that should be first is placed second, that which should be first is not simply demeaned by being demoted to second place, but I is in danger of being either lost or rejected. Placing man ahead of God initially demeans religion, but, as history has shown, leads to a rejection of God. A person who places money above honesty will soon become dishonest. If spouses do not subordinate themselves to each other, their marriage is heading for a separation or divorce.

The great problem in placing the secondary end of sexual intercourse first, is the likelihood that procreation will be demeaned initially and subsequently rejected. But in addition to this, the meaning of lovemaking would inevitably have to be re-invented. Such re-creation would inevitably be arbitrary and therefore subject to a distorted and possibly even perverse interpretation.

The Russian existentialist Nikolai Berdyaev had some insight into this problem when he argued that "If there were no childbearing, sexual union would degenerate into debauchery."[3] Max Horkeimer, the founder of the Frankfurt School of critical social philosophy had a similarly bleak prediction. He prophesied that widespread contraception would destroy romantic love and turn *Romeo and Juliet* into a museum piece. In hindsight, one must acknowledge that these points are well taken. While many have welcomed the "freedom" that contraception offers spouses, a goodly number of them have recognized a need to restore some measure of nobility and romanticism to the sexual act. As insightful an observer of the modern world as the surrealist painter, Salvador Dali, told a *Time* reporter that "The only way to make love is as a sacrament."[4]

Contraception signals the separation of love-making from baby-making. One is left to wonder about the deeper levels of separation that may result: act from meaning, and effort from moral justification.

Man is, according to the precepts of logotherapy, as well as the Judaeo-Christian tradition, a meaning-oriented creature far more than he is a pleasure-seeker. There is no pleasure than man enjoys that he will not ascribe some meaning to it in order to elevate its significance. But the very notion of meaning implies a relationship or correspondence that goes beyond what a thing is in itself. A word has meaning because it is a sign of an intelligibility that transcends the word as such. One is not satisfied in hearing a stream of words; one wants to know what meaning they convey. The activities within a baseball game are meaningful because they are subordinated to the goal of winning. It is the prospect of winning that gives the game its ultimate meaning, otherwise no one would bother to keep score.

Paul Tillich has pointed out that while the great anxiety of antiquity was Death, and the chief anxiety of the Medieval Period was Condemnation, the principal anxiety of the Modern Era is Meaninglessness. This anxiety is a direct result of the fragmentation of the modern world and the preposterousness that results when the natural order of things is reversed. Unable to bear life in a meaningless world, people are compelled to invent meanings. Unfortunately, these fabricated meanings cannot offer real sustenance for human beings. They reduce everything to the status of a game. And while games can be refreshing diversions from the seriousness of life, they cannot nourish the inner spirit that seeks an answer to the question, "What is the meaning of life?" There is an insuppressible kernel of philosophical instinct in all of us that inclines us to search for and be in love with wisdom. In his own self-indulgent way, Alex Comfort is right. The author of the mega-selling secular Bible of sex, *The Joy of Sex*, holds that sex is the most important human sport. But Christopher Derrick is right in an objective way when he states that "The case against *Playboy* and everything similar is that one's attention is thereby fixed not upon sex, but upon sexual unreality."[6]

Fragmentation and preposterousness, therefore, lead to a flight from reality and a preoccupation with fantasy. Reality, of course, being the stronger force, will always be victorious when the two collide. On the dust jacket of a best-selling book that is a panegyric to the revolutionary potential of contraception, we find these words from a mortified young husband: "I married a lovely, sexy girl — then she turned into someone's mother."

People will age and die, beauty will fade, and children will continue to come into the world, planned or unplanned. That is the reality. With the advent of contraception, many actually believed that it would bring about a Paradise on Earth. In the words of one influential feminist, contraception and its kindred technologies "could undo Adam's and Eve's curse both, to reestablish the earthy Garden of Eden."[7]

The Postpill Paradise

The phrase "postpill paradise" belongs to John Updike. It made its first appearance in his novel, *Couples*, which vaulted to the bestseller list within three weeks of publication. The year was 1968, the same year Pope Pius VI issued *Humanae vitae*.

The phrase, of course, is used ironically. The couples who inhabit the novel are obsessed with adultery. They are free, as citizens of the postpill era, to re-invent the meaning of sex. They respond to the challenge with unfettered abandon. For some, adulterous sex is an antidote to boredom, others use it for revenge, and still others to prove that nothing is forbidden to them. They are caught in the exquisite contradiction of playing the role of libertarian hedonists while seeking the joy and meaning of life. Joy, not surprisingly, eludes them. In the book, it has only a nominal existence. It is the name of a creek located in the mythical town of Tarbox, Massachusetts. So, too, are the virtues that could direct the *dramatis personae* to a meaningful existence. "Charity," "prudence," "hope," and "temperance," are the names of streets.

The life of a libertine is a demanding one. When sex means anything one wants it to mean, it becomes highly unlikely that a group of married couples will find their social circle an image of concord and mutual respect. One character alludes to the dilemma when he says: "We're a subversive cell, like in the catacombs. Only they were trying to break out of hedonism. We're trying to break back into it. It's not easy."[8]

The postpill paradise is, needless to say, a nightmare. The novel has an apocalyptic ending, demonstrating that getting what you want does not necessarily mean getting what you need. The undistracted pursuit of pleasure can be an adventure in agonizing futility.

Contracepting the natural end of sexual union and deconstructing its basic nature should leave people not with an exhilarating sense of freedom, but a disturbing sense of meaninglessness. What would the meaning of eating be in the absence of both hunger and nourishment, and the presence of mere will? Dr. Ruth Westheimer, the popular sex education "expert" enjoins people to have "good sex." But all she means by this maxim is high-powered sexual performance. Where does this leave those who are less than sexually athletic? Love, the nature of the relationship, its respect for God's Plan are all neatly factored out of the equation. The performance is the thing. But is this not the ultimate trivialization of sex? If you get a good swing at a baseball late in the game when your team is down by fifteen runs, is the swing of any importance? Bereft of context, drama, and meaning, is it even worth the effort? Other observers of the sex scene were not blind to the fact that what some commentators were calling "liberation," more closely approximated "trivialization." Accordingly, one such observer notes:

> Copulation-centred thought about human sexuality seeks, in the name of liberation, to turn us into sexual virtuosos. 'So and so', we hear people say, 'is good in bed'. Skill in love-making is extremely important to acquire, but when we make it an end in itself and remove the spiritual and total commitment aspects, we relegate sex to the same level as 'she plays a good hand of bridge' or 'he plays a good round of golf'.[9]

The removal of all natural meaning from sexual union cues the introduction of the sex manuals. These "how-to" books are based on the assumption that if there is one thing mates do not know how to do is precisely how to mate. The *Kama Sutra*, *The Joy of Sex*, and other comparable sex-instructions books, are found in plentiful supply in most bookstores. Even when they are not advising excursions in partner-swapping, in accordance with the maxim of Updike's "couples" that the plural of spouse is spice, they may still not be for the faint of heart. As one philosopher warns, "[These] glossy manuals would turn the bedroom into a bordello. A wife is urged to do things that would have brought a blush to the cheek of an experienced courtesan."[10]

The attempt to maximize sex as an end in itself leads logically to its ultimate trivialization. In the game of "trivia", bits of knowledge are considered trivial because they are dissociated from any overriding importance. But if all the importance of sex is compressed into how well it is performed, the inevitable outcome for many people will be what psychologists refer to as "performance anxiety." Impotence and sexual anorexia are also the byproducts of too much emphasis on performance. Sex will be joyful, rather than jaded, when it is accompanied by a rich context of natural and human meanings.

Germain Greer, who once exhorted women to revel in their sexuality, after closely scrutinizing the casualties of the contraceptive revolution, now warns her followers that sex has degenerated into a social gesture that is as trivial as a handshake. She claims that contraceptive technology, instead of liberating women, has turned them into geishas who risk health and fertility in order to be readily available for meaningless sex. Taking the Pill, says Greer, is like "using a steamroller to crush a frog," and the intrauterine device turns the womb into a "poisonous abattoir."[11] A teenage girl with a packet of pills in her purse and a copy of *The Joy of Sex* on her bookshelf is a pitiable creature, according to Greer's new perspective.

Betty Friedan, America's elder stateswoman of feminism, also began singing a different tune to her legion of followers in a book she wrote eighteen years after *The Feminine Mystique*. Having witnessed the negative side of contraception's legacy of "sexual freedom", she used *The Second Stage* to preach the importance of the family, an institution toward, which, she claims, feminists had been "strangely blind." She notes that after two decades of the woman's movement, too many women are facing economic misery as a result of divorce and are devalued in the workplace "and sometimes even replaced by other women who got into the men's world and sometimes took away their husbands."[12] *The Second Stage* redirects the meaning of sex to bolster the relationship between husband and wife so that they are better prepared to be good fathers and mothers. The family, she declares, "is the nutrient of our personhood."[13]

Humanizing Sex

"It seems obvious," writes Dr. Wanda Poltawska, "that the incorrect hierarchy of values grows out of the essence of contraception itself, which calls attention to sex without perceiving the integral value of the human being."[14] The first task of sexual morality, then, is to allow the integral value of the human being to guide us along the path of humanizing sex. This requires a great deal of spiritual insight. For the typical citizen of our contraceptive society, who only too readily reduces relations between the sexes to sexual relations, this is no small challenge.

Henrik Ibsen is Norway's most distinguished dramatist. A man of versatility, his influence as a thinker, in some ways, matched his influence as a playwright. He once stated that "The Bible speaks of a mysterious sin for which there is not forgiveness: this great unpardonable sin is the murder of the 'love-life' in a human being." Putting the question of Scriptural accuracy aside, Ibsen was pointing out that a violation of the natural intimacy between love and life constitutes a most grievous transgression against the Law of God. Love that does not promote life is sterile; to produce life independent of a source of love is blasphemous.

Malcolm Muggeridge, Britain's premier journalist of the twentieth century describes a dramatic "love-life" experience he had with "the person I most loved in this world, my wife Kitty."[15]

Kitty was desperately ill and her attending physician gave her only an outside chance of surviving. An emergency operation was necessary. Before the operation could take place, a blood transfusion was needed because Kitty's blood had been severely thinned as the result of a long spell with jaundice. At the very prospect that he could be the blood donor, "an incredible happiness amounting to ecstasy" surged up within her husband. His blood count was taken and found to be suitable. Husband and wife were then united through a simple glass tube with a pump in the middle, and the health-giving blood began to flow from husband to wife. "Don't stint yourself, take all you want," Muggeridge shouted to the doctor, as he perceived the immediate and salutary effect the gift had in restoring life to her face. It was the turning point; from that moment Kitty began to recover.

Looking back on this incident, Muggeridge write: "At no part in our long relationship has there been a more ecstatic moment than when I thus saw my life-blood pouring into hers to revivify it." To give life is what love is for; its denial is the antithesis of love.

The moment of greatest ecstasy in their long married life, Muggeridge is telling us, was not specifically sexual, but than moment when intimacy between love and life was not only crucial, but transparent. Would it not be ecstatic if spouses could somehow per-ceive God's creation of their new child after the climactic moment of their conjugal embrace? The ecstasy Muggeridge is relating is not the result of sheer physical intensity. It results from a deep and moving experience of the reality of the other person and the inviolable rela-tionship of love and life that binds husband and wife in oneness.

Trying to maximize sexual pleasure would rule out the possibil-ity of ecstasy because the partners are too preoccupied with their own individual satisfactions. In his insightful critique of modern secularism, *Chance or the Dance?* Thomas Howard argues that the void of meaning that plagues the modern world makes ecstasy virtu-ally impossible. The myth sovereign in the old order, he writes, was that each thing *means* everything. The meaning of the sexual act, surely, was not restricted to the mere experience of the act by its per-formers. Accordingly, "a man went in to a woman in private and un-covered her and knew ecstasy in the experience of her being." The myth sovereign in the new order is that "nothing *means* anything."[16] In the new order, we are fragmented, isolated, abandoned, and bereft of ecstasy, despite the exponential multiplication of sex manuals and self-help books.

Sexual morality dwells in the domain of inter-personal reality. It is not concerned primarily with the intensity of a physical experi-ence, but with its *personal quality*. Even a handshake that communi-cates the intimacy of love and life can be more ecstatic than the con-gress of two sexual athletes. An example might help to explain this contention.

At 5:04 p.m. on October 17, 1989, Northern California was rocked by an earthquake that registered 7.1 on the Richter scale. The general public was made instantly aware of this calamity since it was broad-cast "live" for the millions of televiewers who were expecting to watch game three of the World Series between the San Francisco Gi-ants and the Oakland Athletics. The city of San Francisco alone suf-fered billions of dollars in damages; 60 buildings toppled in the Ma-rina district; in Oakland, a mile-and-a-half of Interstate 880's upper roadway buckled; trees writhed and twisted in a windless sky' con-crete walls rippled like tissue paper; automobiles were tossed about like toys. Yet no one could fail to recognize that the greatest loss was registered in human terms — over 70 people were killed, another 1,400 were injured.

The single most dramatic evidence of the earthquake's destruc-tive might was the toppling of the upper roadway on the Nimitz

Freeway. Rescue workers labored around the clock to save whatever victims of the collapsed freeway might still be clinging to life. "The cars up there," exclaimed a shaken rescue worker, "were as flat as their license plates."[17]

As the days passed, hopes of making further rescues began to dim. But the rescue teams worked on, hoping to find some tenacious soul who could outlast all the odds that were stacked against him. And then a riveting story was released over the wire service. A voice had been heard, originating from deep within the rubble. Guided by this sound, rescuers painstakingly cleared away what must have seemed like a lifetime's accumulation of debris until they came to the source of the voice in a trapped automobile. An eager worker reached into the car and grasped the hand of the passenger. The hand squeezed back!

At this point we must allow ourselves the use of a little imagination. Let us cast our trapped passenger in the role of a politician who is heading homeward along the Nimitz Freeway after shaking hands with more strangers than he cares to remember. The handshakes were mechanical, perfunctory, meaningless. He was relieved to get away from the anonymous crowd of annoying well-wishers. But that was his role — to placate his constituency. Then the unexpected happened — the collapse of the upper tier of the freeway, and quite likely, of his life. After that, the endless, anxiety-ridden wait. Jonah in the belly of the whale. A man who shook hands promiscuously was spending what may have been his final hours praying for the touch of a human hand. His prayers were answered. A handshake, the gentlest of tremors, broke into his isolation and reconnected him with human society. It was a handshake that he would set apart from all the other handshakes he would ever receive. It was not the prosaic intersection of self-interest with idle flattery that was his accustomed experience. This handshake was the spiritually charged union of live and life. There was certainly love, a reciprocal love flowing back and forth between the courageous rescuer and the hopeful victim. It was a love that abounded with meaning because it successfully served the life to which it was subordinated.

Let us return now from the realm of the imagination to the world of facts. The news report was not true. The voice that was heard did not come from a live person but from the car radio. The hand squeezed back only in the over-heated imagination of the rescuer. Nonetheless, the story, even though fictional, is still a good one, for it reveals a truth that goes deeper than facts.

The central virtue of the rescue worker, more basic than his courage, hopefulness, and heroic altruism, is his openness to life. The fact that the life he sought no longer existed does not detract a single iota from the value of this virtue. Can we preserve this moral perception as we pass from the realm of heroic rescue operations in the aftermath of an earthquake to the realm of the conjugal embrace? Can we not cherish the notion that spouses who approach each other with the same uncompromising regard for the unity of love and life are any less heroic?

We are creatures who are made for meaning. The shades of boredom quickly descend on the artificial womb that we fabricate out of comfort and security. And what is boredom but the void that results when the dyad of love and life is no longer present?

To humanize sex is to give it its fullness, both with regard to space and time. Sex involves love, life, God, and community; it also has implications of commitment, responsibility, and permanence. Contraception prevents sex from being everything it can and should be. But it also devalues what it excludes, making the process of restoring the integrity of sexual union most difficult. The danger, therefore, perdures, that sexual union will be perceived as trivial *in its essence*. Advocates of contraception initially wanted to improve love-making between spouses. That early optimism is nearly moribund at present. We need to recover something of that optimism. But we cannot expect to restore sexual union to its proper human quality through technology, but only through respecting the values that are inherent in sexuality's immanent and transcendent reality.

Endnotes

[1] Nikolai Berdyaev, *The Meaning of the Creative Act* (New York, NY: Doubleday, 1966), p. 31.

[2] "Allocation to the Roman Rota," *Acta Apostolica Sedis*, 33 (1941), 421-26 at 423.

[3] Nikolai Berdyaev, *The Destiny of Man* (New York, NY: Harper & Row, 1960), p. 242.

[4] As quoted in *Time* [European edition], Nov. 10, 1980, p. 64.

[5] Paul Tillich, *The Courage To Be* (New Haven, CT: Yale University Press, 1965), p. 41.

[6] Christopher Derrick, *Sex and Sacredness* (San Francisco, CA: Ignatius Press, 1982), p. 167.

[7] Shulamith Firestone, *The Dialectic of Sex* (New York, NY: Bantam Books, 1972), p. 211.

[8] John Updike, *Couples* (New York, NY: Alfred Knopf, 1968).

[9] Gavin Reid, *The Elaborate Funeral* (London: Hodden & Stoughton, 1972), p. 109.

[10] Ralph McInerny, "The Domestication of Hedonism," *Catholic Dossier*, Vol. 3, No. 5, Sept.-Oct. 1997, p. 7.

[11] Gillian MacKay, "Life With Less Sex," *Maclean's* April 16, 1984, p. 40.

[12] Betty Friedan, *The Second Stage* (New York, NY: Summit Books, 1981), p. 83.

[13] *Ibid.*, p. 99.

[14]Wanda Poltawska, "The Effect of a Contraceptive Attitude on Marriage," *The International Review of Natural Family Planning*, Vol. IV, No. 3, Fall 1980, p. 191.

[15]Malcolm Muggeridge, "The Human Holocaust," in Ronald Reagan, *Abortion and the Conscience of a Nation* (Nashville, TN: Nelson, 1984), pp. 92-3.

[16]Thomas Howard, *Chance or the Dance?* (San Francisco, CA: Ignatius Press, 1969), pp. 12-3.

[17]Scot Haller *et al.*, "A City Trembled, Its People Held," *People,* Oct. 30, 1989, pp.34-6.

Contraception as a Gateway to Abortion

Contraception is the practice of using any mechanical or chemical means whose purpose is to insure that sexual intercourse does not result in conception. Abortion (that is, direct, induced abortion) is the deliberate expulsion of a pre-natal human being from his mother's womb, an act that almost always results in his death. Contraception prevents life from coming into being; abortion destroys a life that is already present. Contraception and abortion are distinct acts and have distinct moral implications. In fact, many people are convinced that they are actually antagonistic to each other. Contraception, it is believed, reduces the need for abortion; too easy access to abortion discourages the use of contraception. Many people, therefore, approve contraception precisely because they oppose abortion.

It is not surprising, then, that a vast body of responsible social agencies have zealously promoted the use of contraception as a way of lowering the incidence of abortion. It is equally not surprising that these same agencies could not begin to understand why the Catholic Church, that opposed abortion, would also oppose contraception, the ostensive preventative of abortion. Typical of this attitude is a statement issued by the religion editor of Canada's most widely circulated newspaper:

> Surely to oppose abortion on the one hand while on the other fiercely opposing sex education and the very contraceptives which could prevent unwanted pregnancies, as many religious groups of varying persuasion do, seems an illogical — and often tragic — mistake.[1]

The Rule of Plausibility

H. L. Mencken once said that there is a solution for everything that is neat, plausible, and wrong. Research has demonstrated beyond doubt that the plausible hypothesis that more contraception would lead to less abortion is untenable. Kristin Luker's book, *Taking Chances: Abortion and the Decision Not to Contracept*, supplied the most compelling documentation that had been provided up to that time (1975) that explained why women who did not want to get pregnant frequently chose not to contracept. Luker, a sociologist at the University of California in San Diego, was well aware that her findings challenged the "rules of plausibility", as she admitted. No longer intellectually able to separate contraception from abortion in the moral choices of women, she concluded that the failure of contraception necessitated the full acceptance of abortion:

> We would argue that since abortion has become a primary method of fertility control, it should be offered in exactly the same way that the other contraceptive services are.[2]

Luker found abundant evidence that, given all the personal, emotional, medical, and psychological "costs" of contraception, it was entirely rational for a woman to shun contraception and risk an unwanted pregnancy. She implored society to recognize that a woman who does not want to get pregnant is not behaving irrationally if she does not use contraception while being sexually active. She asked society to be more understanding of such women and allow them the privilege of defining their own situation.[3]

The year after Luker's study was published, a government sponsored publication in Canada, *Birth Control and Abortion*, presented abortion as an inevitable adjunct to failed contraception:

> As long as contraception methods are not 100% effective and safe, and as long as women wish to control their fertility, requests for abortion can be expected to continue . . . . Today abortion is the most widely used birth-control method in the world.[4]

The following year, the Canadian government's *Badgley Report* showed that 84% of women who had abortions were experienced in using contraception. By 1982, given the considerable costs associated with contraception, the United States government required that each Pill package come with a detailed two-page insert that spells out the dangers of the Pill in easy-to-understand language and describes various contraceptive alternatives. Significantly, it included a chart showing that the barrier methods — backed up by abortion in the event of failure — posed the fewest "health risks" for all age groups.[5]

At the 1982 annual meeting of the National Abortion Foundation, Philip Lee, M. D. predicted that in the coming years, 50 to 60% of all abortions would be performed on repeat clients. In addition, he stated that even "consistent use of contraceptive methods considered most reliable produces not insignificant failure rates."[6] Biostatistician Christopher Tietze calculated that 2-5% of women using the Pill with a reasonable degree of motivation would be likely to have a repeat abortion within a year of their first abortion, and, within ten years of their first abortion, between 20-50% of Pill users may be expected to experience at least one other unplanned pregnancy.[7]

Professors John Kantner and Melvin Zelnik of Johns Hopkins University did three separate national surveys of sexual activity, contraceptive use, pregnancy, and abortion among American teenage girls. These surveys, all similar, were carried out in 1971, 1976, and 1979. Their results confirmed the increasingly well-established conclusion that contraception is linked with abortion.

The research showed that out-of-wedlock births rose from 190,000 in 1970 to 240,000 in 1979, while the number of abortions grew from 90,000 to 500,000, and the number of unintended pregnancies rose steadily from 8.5% in 1970 to 13% in 1976 to 16.2% in 1979. Concurrent with these increases of out-of wedlock pregnancies, abortions, and unintended pregnancies was an increased use of contraception. The number who always used contraception was 20% greater in 1979 than in 1976, while the number who never contracepted during this period dropped by about 25%. Most startling, perhaps, especially for those who believed in the plausible hypothesis that a greater use of contraception means a smaller rate of abortion, was the fact that almost one-third (31.5%) of the unintended pregnancies in 1979 occurred while a contraceptive method was in use, a proportion almost four times as high as the 1971 figure of 8.6%. And nearly half the unintended premarital pregnancies (49.7%) occurred among young women who had used a contraceptive at some time. Moreover, Kantner and Zelnik discovered that teenage girls who became pregnant while using contraception were twice as likely to seek an abortion as those who became pregnant in the absence of contraception.

Unintended pregnancies and abortions increased significantly among teenagers despite their using more effective forms of contraception and employing them more frequently and more regularly. Part of the explanation of this paradox lies in the fact that the incidence of teenage intercourse rose to a level that offset whatever advantage contraception may have represented. Indeed, the increase in premarital sex was so great that it surpassed the limits of effectiveness birth control and abortion clinics provided in an attempt to hold down the number of out-of-wedlock births.

Michael Schwartz and James Ford, M. D., who carefully analyzed the Kantner-Zelnik survey concluded that "it is clear that the family planning programs have contributed directly to an increase in the rate of abortion among teenagers." In providing teenagers with a program of contraception and tacitly encouraging them to engage in sexual intercourse, family programs in the United States not only failed to realize their objectives, but brought on more of the disease. In the words of Schwartz and Ford, it proved a "diagram for disaster."[8]

All of the above studies have corroborated what was foreshadowed in earlier, more limited studies. In England, for example, the Royal Commission on Population noted that in 1949 the number of procured abortions was 8.7 times higher among couples who habitually practiced contraception than among those who did not. In Sweden, after contraception had been fully legalized, legal abortions increased from 703 in 1943 to 6,328 in 1951. In Switzerland, where contraception was almost unrestricted, abortions were alleged to equal or outnumber live births by 1955, and so on.[9] Such figures offer compelling evidence that increased contraception does not reduce the incidence of abortion. Rather, contraception tends to establish a *contraceptive mentality* that leads to absolving responsibility for children conceived, which, in turn, leads to *more* abortion.

The story is told of a team of fishermen that was concerned about its dwindling clam harvest. When the fishermen realized that their crop was being ravaged by starfish, they applied a plausible solution to the problem by hauling the predators onto their boats, chopping them in half, and tossing the severed remains back into the sea. Yet they were astonished to discover that the more starfish they bisected, the more clams they lost. Their critical error was their failure to understand how their enemy operated. Starfish have the capacity to regenerate. By cutting them in half, the fishermen were doubling their population. In effect, they had been engaged in the embarrassing plight of fighting against themselves.

The Contraceptive Mentality

The "contraceptive mentality" is a state of mind characterizing those people who believe that their "responsible" use of contraception entitles them to be free from the burden of an unwanted baby. Contraception is the rejection of the unwanted child in theory, abortion is its rejection in practice. The contraceptive mentality is the frame of mind that united practice with theory. Philosopher Joseph Boyle explains:

> . . .the approval of contraception leads — though not in such a direct and logical way — to acceptance of abortion. Contracep-

tion is an attempt to prevent the handing on of life, and one who turns against life as it is passed on is likely to remain against it if the unwanted new life begins. The resolve to prevent a child from coming to be is often sufficiently strong that one will eliminate the child whose conception was not prevented. This anti-life attitude is often regarded as a "responsible" stance; it often includes the denial that human life is a basic good and the determination that one can do whatever is necessary to execute one's resolve to prevent a person from coming to be.[10]

As early as the 1930's, historian Christopher Dawson had expressed the fear that widespread contraception would be a threat to marriage. He urged people to re-spiritualize sexuality in order to preserve its true meaning.[11] Dawson was accused at that time of being an alarmist for expressing such a view. Also in the 1930's, Dr. Paul Popenoe complained, in his book, *Modern Marriage*, of real difficulties in marriage that were "intensified by an emotional propaganda, much of which was associated with the earlier years of the birth-control movement." He went on to say:

> For well over a quarter century, America was assailed with propaganda painting the evils of large families, the dangers of child-bearing, the misfortunes of the 'unwanted child' (without taking much trouble to inquire why he was unwanted). . . . From a good deal of modern discussion one would think that children were a misfortune; that the smallest number was a desirable number, that each additional child was for the mother a step toward the grave, for father a step toward bankruptcy, and for both a step toward misery.

The first person to draw attention specifically to a "contraceptive mentality" and offer statistical evidence to support its widespread existence, was the Jesuit sociologist Stanislas de Lestapis. In his book, *La limitation des naissances*, published in 1960, de Lestapis provided sociological data that indicated the presence of what he termed a "contraceptive state of mind."[12]

At the heart of the "contraceptive mentality" is the notion that the unwanted child is an evil. This seems to be the logical outcome of regarding contraception as positive. Because contraception is presumed to be positive, the thing it keeps away, the unwanted child, must be cast in a negative light. The unwanted child, as it were, has no business coming into being when the contracepting couple made it only too clear that they did not want him. The well has been poisoned, and when a child comes into existence in a contraceptive atmosphere, he is likely to remain as unwelcome in practice as he was in theory. A former Supreme Court Justice has expressed the matter rather succinctly: "If an individual may prevent conception, why can he not nullify that conception when prevention has failed?"[13] And a prominent sociologist states that "this is probably the first generation in the history of mankind which is being told that the child itself is the evil, and a menace to the human race."[14]

The anti-baby root of the "contraceptive mentality" was brought home in an unexpected way a few years ago when G. D. Searle and Company was trying to market its anovulent contraceptive in Turkey. The chief obstacle it ran into was that there was no word for contraception in the Turkish language. The Pill was eventually marketed to the Turkish people under the equivalent of the "have no baby" pill. A more direct illustration of the anti-baby essence of the "contraceptive mentality" is offered by Montreal's Dr. Lise Fortier. At a meeting of the National Abortion Federation, Dr. Fortier told her audience that "each and every pregnancy threatens a woman's life" and that from a strict medical viewpoint "every pregnancy should be aborted."[15] On a more casual level, zero-populationist Ellen Peck informed her readers that "if birth control has been neglected or has failed; and if the morning after [pill] has passed; there is the option of an abortion."[16]

According to Pope John Paul II, the "contraceptive mentality" strengthens the temptation to abort the child that was initially unwanted. He also points out that "the pro-abortion culture is especially strong precisely where the Church's teaching on contraception is rejected."[16] Despite the negative values inherent in the contraceptive mentality, a certain sense of righteousness prevails. When people ascribe the virtue of responsibility to their deliberate employment of contraception, they often feel that they do not deserve to be punished by taking on the obligation of delivering and caring for a child they never wanted. This contraceptive attitude has been encouraged and reinforced systematically through well organized political and cultural forces.

Promoting the Contraceptive Mentality

In his study of the history of the birth control movement in American society, author James Reed maintains that the major obstacle to wider acceptance of contraception was less technological than psychological. Similarly, he argues that the development of the Pill and other contraceptive devices owed more to changes in social values than to technological opportunity. This psychological barrier was overcome primarily by the effect of intense and relentless propaganda. But the leading propagandists carefully avoided or suppressed the fact that contraception contains an implication of abortion. This they revealed only at such time when the public was ready to accept abortion on its own.

In the United States, two very powerful organizations, the American Civil Liberties Union (ACLU) and the Planned Parenthood Federation (PPF) worked hand in glove to establish the "right" to contraception, which became law in 1965.[18] Working together, they helped establish the contraceptive mentality as an important feature of the American way of life. Significantly, both groups ostensibly viewed abortion as an undesirable objective. They predicted that an increase in contraceptive practice would result in a decrease in abortions. But their public campaign to promote contraception were kept free of any endorsement of abortion, not because their leaders opposed abortion but because the public was not ready for pro-abortion propaganda.

Margaret Sanger, the foundress of Planned Parenthood in the United States, had condoned abortion in her 1916 edition of *Family Limitation*, stating that "No one can doubt that abortion is justifiable."[19] But her colleague, Havelock Ellis, helped persuade her to change her public stance on the matter, shrewdly advising her that the "right to create or not create new life" had better propaganda value than the "right to destroy." As a result, Mrs. Sanger began using abortion as a lever to make contraception more acceptable, arguing that contraception would put an end to abortion. Abortions are "barbaric," she then exclaimed, though disingenuously, and classified it with infanticide as "the killing of babies."[20]

As later as 1961, Alan Guttmacher, president of Planned Parenthood in the United States, wrote concerning the origin of human life: "Fertilization, then, has taken place; a baby has been conceived."[21] This remark was consistent with an observation he had made in an earlier work, *Having a Baby* (1947), where he referred to the being who was produced by fertilization as "the new baby which is created at this exact moment." But in 1968, when he was international president, the time was ripe for endorsing abortion; consequently, he changed his tactics and declared that "My feeling is that the fetus, particularly during its intrauterine life, is merely a group of specialized cells that do not differ materially from other cells."[22]

The contraceptive mentality contained the seeds of the abortion mentality. But certain morally revolutionary events were needed in order to prepare the ground for public acceptance of abortion. These events were mainly four. The first was connected with the moral and ideological turmoil of the 1960's which led to a rethinking (some would call it a "doing away with thinking") of traditional views of sexual morality. The other three were more specific: the rise of feminism, the recognition of the hazards of the Pill, and the appearance of anxious world population watchers monitoring the "population explosion."

The feminist movement which put forward a view of women's liberation that included the right to abortion had a decisive impact on the ACLU. As a result of feminist influence, the ACLU adopted a pro-abortion stance and dispatched its best constitutional lawyer, Norman Dorsen, to the appeal of *Roe v. Wade* in the United States Supreme Court which was to legalize abortion on demand for the first trimester.[23] The well publicized news of the dangers of the oral contraceptive led many to abandon the "ideal contraceptive" and either resort to lesser effective contraceptive measures or assume the risk of an unwanted pregnancy. The so-called "population explosion" gave rise to a panic rhetoric that was largely accepted without question by the media. All four events are intricately interwoven. The rejection of traditional values was largely a preference to separate sex from marriage, children, and religious dogma, that is, to make sex more "personal" or, in the language of the courts, more "private." This preference was congenial to feminists who were demanding a liberation from all traditional expectations or values, and one that would be interpreted purely according to the prerogatives of the individual women themselves. The need for an effective and safe contraceptive was a crucial and obvious step along this road to personal and sexual liberation. It may be observed that the United States Supreme Court decision, *Griswald v. Connecticut*, established the right to contraception on the basis of the right to privacy. Thus it offered the philosophical basis in *Roe v. Wade* in 1973 to legitimize abortion on demand in the first trimester. Writing for the Court, Justice Douglas wrote: "We deal with a right to privacy older than the Bill of Rights — older than our political parties, older than our school system."

The Pill was also viewed as a way of solving the "population crisis" and this fact shaped the minds of people who were influential in approving the Pill for widespread distribution. Louis Hellman, chairman of the Food and Drug Administration's Advisory Committee on Obstetrics and Gynecology interpreted the law to permit the Pill's distribution — despite warning from the scientific community that it was not safe for some women — by balancing the *social* against the risk to the *individual*. Hellman testified before a Congressional Hearing on "Oral Contraceptives" (Jan. 22, 1970) that he had associated himself with the Administration because "the threat of population growth" was "real to each and every individual of this country." Nevertheless, the Pill, which produced diseased conditions in millions of women, proved not to be the ally it was presumed to be in the feminists' quest for liberation.

The promoters of the contraceptive mentality were not about to back down when signs of contraceptive failure appeared everywhere. Failure seemed to arouse in them only a greater commitment to the very principles that brought about such disappointing consequences. In response to this, Planned Parenthood vice-president Frederick Jaffe declared: "To cope with this epidemic we need new conception control methods more effective and acceptable than the Pill and higher program priority and greater resources for biomedical research." The new forms of conception control, however, would inevitably mean abortion on a greater scale than ever before.

The Effects of the Contraceptive Mentality

The "contraceptive mentality", which begins in the dissociation of intercourse from conception, logically and inevitably results in the dissociation of conception from life. As Malcolm Potts, the former medical director of the International Planned parenthood Federation, accurately predicted in 1973: "As people turn to contraception, there will be a rise, not a fall, in the abortion rate."[24] It was an easy prediction to make in the light of what had transpired in other countries.

There is virtual universal agreement that abortion is highly undesirable. But repeatedly, as shown above, opponents of abortions who are themselves victims of the contraceptive mentality defend the indefensible thesis that contraception will reduce abortion.

Historically, the explanation seems obvious. As contraception received a "green light", the number of abortions increased. Wherever the contraceptive mentality prevailed, abortion was the logical outcome of contraceptive failure. Therefore, in countries that accepted contraception for general use, the increasing number of abortions compelled authorities to make them legal. This second "green light", escalated the number of abortions to tens of millions throughout the world every year.

Pope John Paul II was understating the matter when he wrote: "The close connection which exists in mentality, between the practice of contraception and that of abortion is becoming increasingly obvious."[25] Less understated is the remark of a prominent Catholic philosopher: "The link between contraception and abortion is now clear to all."[26]

A survey released in 1996 by the Alan Guttmacher Institute shows that between 1994 and 1995, 57.5% of 10,000 abortion patients were using contraception during the month in which they became pregnant, up from 51.3% who answered a similar query in the late 1980's.[27] And a medical advisor for Planned Parenthood reports that "More than three million unplanned pregnancies occur each year to American women; two-thirds of these are due to contraceptive failure."[28]

The contraceptive mentality has unified contraception and abortion so tightly that abortion is commonly referred to as a form of contraception. The contraception euphemisms used to describe abortion are numerous: "your second chance to practice contraception," "post-coital fertility control," "post-conception contraception," "the morning-after *Pill*," and "emergency contraception."

That contraception is a gateway to abortion has been established beyond any reasonable doubt. Both contraception and abortion share an anti-life frame of mind. It should be evident that fighting abortion is short-sighted if one does not recognize its roots in the contraceptive mentality. From a historical perspective, it has not been possible to prevent contraception from giving rise to abortion. Contraception does not prevent abortion; it is simply a more subtle form of opposing life.

Endnotes

[1] Tom Harpur, *Toronto Star*, June 12, 1982.

[2] Kristin Luker, *Taking Chances: Abortion and the Decision Not to Contracept* (Berkeley, CA: University of California Press, 1975), p. 144.

[3] *Ibid.*, p. 17.

[4] Robertson *et al. Sex Education: a teacher's guide, published by the authority of The Minister of Natural Health and Welfare*, vol. 4, pp. 74-5.

[5] Linda McQuaig, "Living without the Pill," *Maclean's*, March 15, 1982, p. 45.

[6] Andrew Scholberg, "Abortionists Meet: 1982," *Life and Family News*, June-July, 1982, p. 1.

[7] Cited by Paul Marx, "Theological Tomfoolery and Contraception," *Restoration*, Feb. 1979.

[8] M. Schwartz and J. Ford, "Birth Control for Teenagers: Diagram for Disaster," *Linacre Quarterly*, Feb. 1979.

[9] John Noonan, Jr., *Contraception: A History of its Treatment by the Catholic Theologians and Canonists* (New York, NY: American Library, 1965), p. 614.

[10] Joseph Boyle, "Contraception and Natural Family Planning," *International Review of Natural Family Planning*, Vol. Iv, No. 4, Winter 1980, pp. 311-12.

[11] Christopher Dawson, *Enquiries into Religion and Culture* (1933). See *The Dawson Newsletter*, Vol. 1, No. 2, Fall 1981.

[12]Stanislas de Lestapis, S. J., *La limitation des naissances*, 2nd. ed. (Paris, 1960), pp. 64-5.

[13]Tom Clark, *Loyola University of Los Angeles Law Review* (2, No. 1, 1969).

[14]James Schall, S. J., *Human Dignity and Human Numbers* (New York, NY: Allba House, 1971), pp. 67, 78.

[15]Andrew Scholberg, "The Abortionists and Planned Parenthood: Familiar Bedfellows," *International Review of Natural Family Planning*, Vol. IV, No. 4, Winter 1980, p. 308.

[16]Ellen Peck, *The Baby Trap* (New York, NY: Geis Associates, 1971), p. 151.

[17]John Paul II, *Evangelium Vitae*, sec. 13.

[18]The United States Supreme Court Decision, *Griswold v. Connecticut*.

[19]Elasah Drogin, *Margaret Sanger: Father of Modern Society* (Coarsegold, CA: CUL Publications, 1979), p. 69.

[20]Margaret Sanger, *My Fight for Birth Control* (New York, NY: Farrar & Rinehart, 1931), p. 133.

[21]Alan F. Guttmacher, *Birth Control and Love: The Complete Guide to Contraception and Fertility* (New York, NY: Macmillan, 1961), p. 12.

[22]Alan F. Guttmacher, "Symposium: Law, Morality, and Abortion," *Rutgers Law Review* 22 (1960): 415-16.

[23]John Noonan, Jr., *A Private Choice* (New York, NY: Macmillan, 1979), p. 36.

[24]Scholberg, *op. cit.* 1980, p. 298.

[25]John Paul II, *op. cit.*

[26]Ralph McInerny, *op. cit.*, p. 9.

[27]*Human Life International Special Report No. 142*, Oct. 1996, p. 10.

[28]Louise Tyler, *Wall Street Journal*, April 26, 1991.

Contraception and Being a Person

Contraception is a moral issue. It is also a religious issue. But it is possible, setting religion aside, to analyze and discuss the issue of contraception strictly on a natural level. Moral philosophers are concerned with ordinary and natural experiences of all human beings. They develop their discipline by using reason, a universal human possession, to illuminate why certain acts are good for human beings and why other acts are not. A moral analysis of contraception, then, is equally relevant to Protestants, Jews, Moslems, Hindi, and atheists, as well as Catholics. In order to begin distinguishing between what acts are good and what acts are not good for human beings, it is first necessary to respond to the question, "What does it mean to be a human being?" This question, essentially anthropological in nature, must be dealt with before one is in a position to go on and deal with the more specific issues involving the moral implications that contraceptive acts have for human beings, marriage, and society.

The Human Being as a Person

There is a journal that is published under the title, *Conscience, "A News Journal of Prochoice Catholic Opinion"* which is devoted to moral issues such as contraception. This journal reflects the popular and commonly held opinion that no authority, other than one's own conscience, has the right to dictate personal moral choices to anyone. Contraception is a matter that should be left to the conscience of the individual.

This popular and commonly held view of conscience is false even to the meaning of the word "conscience." Etymologically, the word "conscience" (in Latin < *con* + *scientia*) literally means *with knowledge*. One's conscience cannot be formed in an intellectual void. Conscience, to be properly formed, requires knowledge. Similarly, *choice* is not truly a choice in the absence of knowledge. A choice without knowledge is more accurately a "stab in the dark" or "a wild guess." The fact that there is no group that declares itself to be "pro-stab-in-the-dark" or "pro-guess" is not without importance. Choice, like conscience, must be enlightened, if it is to have the possibility of functioning in a way that is beneficial to the individual. In other words, conscience and choice are not functional unless they are enlightened by knowledge. This enlightenment is precisely what moral philosophers seek to provide.

Conscience is enfeebled when it is divorced from truth (or knowledge of what is true). At the same time, when conscience possesses truth, freedom is not compromised in the process. Conscience, truth, and freedom all thrive, so to speak, in each other's presence. One freely chooses to act in a certain way because his informed conscience tells him that it is the right way to act. If I know that a medicinal I had intended to give my wife is actually poisonous to her, given her condition, I will freely choose not to give it to her. I will not regard my knowledge as a source of authoritarianism; nor will I conclude that by deciding wholeheartedly to act one way and not the other, I forfeited my freedom. Truth, freedom, and conscience are mutual allies. To isolate conscience from this triad of life, is to contradict its essential operation. Conscience alone is most unhelpful.

This triad of truth, freedom, and conscience furnishes us with a most important insight into the nature of the human being. It indicates that a human being is not merely an individual who is free to do as he pleases, but is a communal being who is, from the very core of his being, related to a world around him which he can know, and to other human beings whom he can love. Conscience is his inclination to do good and to avoid evil; knowledge is what enlightens his conscience; love is his free choice to serve the good of others.

It is instructive to recall that Pope Paul VI's Majority Report, that urged him to approve the use of contraception for Catholic couples in some instances, remained strong in its opposition to the vices of "egocentricity" and "hedonism." Even here we find a sense that the human being is not a mere individual, an island entity, but a person who, by nature and destiny, is called to take his place in the community of other human beings.

It is also instructive to recall that various Catholic bishops responded to *Humanae Vitae* by placing a disproportionate amount of emphasis on conscience, thereby virtually de-emphasizing the role of knowledge, especially knowledge of the nature of the human being and the nature of sexual union. This, no doubt, left many of the faithful with the impression that conscience may function, somehow, independently of knowledge. A few examples: "Pastors must respect the responsible decisions of conscience made by the faithful" (German bishops); "No one should be considered a bad Catholic because he is of such a dissenting opinion" (Scandinavian bishops); "[There are] many factors which determine one's personal conscience regarding marriage rules, for examples, mutual love, the relations in a family, and social circumstances" (Dutch bishops); "[W]hoever honestly chooses that course which seems right to him does so in good conscience" (Canadian bishops).

Jacques Maritain, one of the foremost personalist philosophers of the twentieth century states that man "superexists" through knowledge and love.[1] Accordingly, the human *person* superexists in knowledge by what he receives through the intellect, and superesists in love by what he gives through the will. René Descartes, the 16th century rationalist philosopher, portrayed man in radically different terms. The "Father of Modern Philosophy", whose influence on modern consciousness cannot be underestimated, depicted man as an isolated and disembodied creature. His timeless proclamation, "I think therefore I am," implied that man is not a person, a communal being, but essentially a thinker, and one who, strangely enough, is alienated from his own body.

While the Majority Report rejected selfish individualism, it did not entirely reject the Cartesian dualism that divorced body from soul. It allowed contraception to negate the body's role in conception so that lovemaking could express "a legitimate communication of persons." But its concept of "person" was more that of a soul that was freed from the generative potential of the body.

It is within the framework of the human person that Pope John Paul II states that *"body and soul are inseparable*: in the person, in the willing agent and in the deliberate act *they stand or fall together."*[2] The person is an inviolable unity. To denigrate one part or the other is not compatible with affirming his status as a person. To approve the use of contraception on the basis that the spiritual love which husband and wife express to each other in sexual intercourse is superior to their bodily or physical integrity, exemplifies a violation of this personal unity.

We are not souls who have bodies. We are beings, that is persons, who express ourselves through our bodies. The body is not an instrument, but an integral part of our being as human persons. Our dignity is in our wholeness. To strike against our wholeness, which contraception does, is to strike against our dignity.

False Images of the Person

The word "person", as commonly used in contemporary society, does not begin to convey the richness that exists within the actual human person, or the richness of meaning it contains in the literature of personalism. It is commonly employed as a synonym for the *individual*. In some cases it represents a self-centered individual, in other cases it appears to be a terrible weight from which individuals seek deliverance.

A medical doctor has proposed a "Personal Marriage Contract" for the modern couple, which is presumed to be a breakthrough of sorts, that truly honors the personalities of husband and wife. One does not need to read very far into this contract before it becomes apparent that it was conceived with self-centered individuals in mind. A sampler of its stipulations are as follows: "I accept my ultimate aloneness and responsibility for myself. . . . I will put myself first. By keeping myself full, satisfied and not hungry, I will have an abundance of joy, love and caring to give you. . . . Don't expect me to accept you as you are when you fail to maintain physical attractiveness, and fail to take care of your body. . . I will not diminish you by thinking of you as 'the wife' or 'the husband'."[3]

By contrast, novelist Gore Vidal believes that having a personality is rather oppressive. He finds that sex is a convenient way to get away from it, even though only momentarily. For Vidal, sex allows couples to upgrade their personalities to "thinghood." "Sex that makes a thing of the partner is a joy," he writes. "There is nothing more depressing to any of us than our personalities. . . . I say, 'The best thing a person can be is a thing.' And two things meeting consensually is what it's all about."[4]

Psychologist Paul Vitz has done an extensive study on how the word "person" is used within his own discipline. What psychologists often mean by "person", he contends, is, in reality, the reduced notion of an individual. "This means," he writes, "that when Carl Rogers titles his best known book, 'On Becoming a Person', he is simply wrong. Instead, what Rogers wrote was a book about becoming an individual — an autonomous, self-actualizing individual who is devoted to the growth of the secular self. But he is not talking about a *person*."[5]

The meaning of "person", in the contemporary world, is also very much tied to capitalism and consumerism. Man is *Homo economicus* or *Homo consumens*. Such false notions of the person lend themselves to strong arguments in favor of the use of contraception. It seems coldly impersonal to discourage a married couple that is struggling economically and cannot afford another child from using contraception. But the true personal dimension of the human being is not understood in terms of economic activity. Married couples should make prudent choices about family size, and their financial situation is most relevant to this kind of decision-making. But they must not ignore their reality as persons. They must not ignore the effect that contraception might have on their personal integrity, their capacity for generous love, and the intimacy quality of their marital relationship. Natural family planning is at least as effective a method of regulating family size and the spacing of children. And it does not infringe upon or compromise their integrity as persons.

The many false notions of what it means to be a person that are promulgated by the media, popular psychology, and the market place, make it particularly difficult for people to understand how anyone could find contraception morally objectionable. Contraception, nonetheless, is inconsistent with the high degree of authentic personhood that marriage demands. Marriage is above all else a communion of persons. It cannot abide being anything less than that.

Personhood and Marriage

The Woman without a Shadow (Die Frau ohne Schatten), by Richard Strauss, is probably the only major opera in which the issue of contraception plays an important role. In addition to contraception, the story-line of the opera illustrates, in a manner that is both fanciful and philosophically sound, the nuptial significance of the body and the personal meaning of marriage.

The story begins when the Emperor traps what appears to be a gazelle. His quarry is really the daughter of a spirit-king, a magical fairy who has the power to transform herself into any shape she desires. As the Emperor is about to drive his spear into her, she changes into a woman of such spellbinding beauty that he immediately falls in love with her and demands that she become his wife.

As the plot develops, the Empress finds herself in a tragic dilemma. If she fails to conceive a child by her husband before the twelfth moon, the Emperor will be turned to stone. She is unable to conceive because, being spiritual in her essence, she does not have a body. She is, in fact, a "crystal soul." In order to conceive, she must involve herself in a maneuver that sets up another dilemma. She must obtain a shadow from a woman who is willing to surrender it, and along with it, her claim to her own future children. The shadow symbolizes the power to conceive, since a child, being cast in the same form as the body from which it came, is in a sense a shadow.

The Empress finds a poor woman who is ready to barter away her future offspring for the comfort and security, riches and earthly glory that her enchanted benefactor can grant her. At the same time, she is conscience-stricken by the impending barter. She listens anxiously and attentively to the mournful sounds of her unborn children who sing to her:

> Mother, Mother, let us come home!
> The door is bolted, we cannot get in.[6]

Her children are, in effect, contracepted by their mother's avarice. Yet, the Empress is also gravely troubled. The realization that she would be robbing this woman and her husband of what would be their greatest treasure, their own children, affects her greatly and is instrumental in helping her to acquire compassion and a conscience. She begins to rue her decision to cheat this married couple of their children in order to obtain her shadow. As a result of her self-forgetful concern for others, a disposition that is the essence of love, she is transformed. She is now worthy of becoming a true human being, obtains a body, in effect, and becomes pregnant.

The tragic dilemmas in the opera are resolved through the intervention of a higher power. The Empress appeals to her father, the spirit-king, who grants his daughter a shadow and removes the curse or petrifaction that threatened her husband. The opera closes happily and triumphantly as the chorus of unborn children sing, assuaging their parents' fears while joyfully anticipating their eventual arrival in the world. They are the reward for their parents who were loyal to them to the point of self-denial.

Die Frau is telling us that it is only in the unity of love and life that happiness can be found and disaster avoided. On the one hand, love without life produces petrifaction, an appropriate symbol of the hardness that results form not giving. On the other hand, life without love represents a certain cold-heartedness, a disregard for the welfare of others. As is the case in much of German romanticism, the integration of love and life is achieved through divine intervention. This is equivalent to saying that the synthesis of life and love reflects the mind and heart of God.

Some psychiatric researchers, after studying the effects of contraception on marriage have come to the conclusion that the contraceptive attitude "destroys love, leads to unfaithfulness, and causes disintegration of the marriage."[7] They have also reported that it "destroys the couple's psychic life."[8] These findings should not be surprising inasmuch as contraception represents a divided and therefore inconstant allegiance between the spouses.

If partners can sometimes compromise, by using contraception, the integrity of their sexual relationship within marriage, why should they not be able to make a similar compromise outside of marriage? Why should cheating within marriage not lead to cheating outside of marriage? Is it not unrealistic to expect that sexually active adults will always remain faithful to their spouses? The logic of contraception provides marital partners with good reason to be anxious and uncertain about the stability of their marriage. A strong case can be made that there is a direct connection between the use of contraception and contemporary culture's high rate of divorce.[9]

We are often far more sensitive to the dark side of our human nature than to its bright side (if we can call it that). We easily forgive moral transgressions on the basis that, after all, "we are only *human*." "Well, what do you expect," we say with stoic resignation? "It's *human nature*." We commonly regard our own nature not only as our worst enemy, but an incorrigible one. It is often easier for us, therefore, to rationalize the use of contraception than to see its dangers. The "bright" side, that is, the uncorrupted side of our human nature, though not as importunate as its darker counterpart, tells us who we are as persons. And as we get in touch with the personal center of our being, we discover that it is a core of generosity.

Personhood and Generosity

Marriage, by nature, is a communion of persons, as we have mentioned. As persons, the spouses honor each other's body/soul unity and also love each other, for love is the most appropriate way of responding to another person. This is what has been referred to as the "intra-conjugal" dimension of marriage. Overriding this horizontal dimension is the "trans-conjugal" that extends to the conception, begetting, care, and education of their children. This is the vertical dimension of their marital relationship. The natural ordering of the two persons in marriage to each other and then, as a married couple to their children (and, possibly, to their children's children), is testimony of the unfolding generosity that originates in the core of their being and characterizes their life as a whole. Paradoxically, in giving to each other, the lives of husband and wife expand into an ever widening community.

Becoming fixated at the level of individuality does not reveal the generous core of one's personhood. When G. K. Chesterton remarked that "Sex is an instinct that produces an institution," he was offering a thumbnail sketch of the social evolution of the human person.[10] The institution to which he refers is marriage and the family. The evolution that takes place is from isolated individualism to a mature human community. Sex is the gateway; the institution is the house. Some people seem to prefer spending their lives hanging around the gateway and not bother to enter the house. Man is a transcendent being. He is called to live generously and move up to higher ground. Too much preoccupation with sex is like spending one's lifetime at the gate and not getting on with one's life. Man is called to transcendence, but his response is often lethargic.

The notion of a hierarchy is not very fashionable in today's world. Equality is in; hierarchy is out. Notions of generosity, growth, personhood, and evolution all imply a hierarchy so that they can advance along their vertical axes. Absolute equality is a flattened, purely horizontal world, one in which personality cannot possibly develop.

Aristotle talked about a natural hierarchy that exists between "the end of the worker" (*finis operantis*) and "the end of the work" (*finis operis*). A soldier, according to Aristotle, enjoys a number of remunerations for his work as a soldier. Among these would be salary, respect, and honor. The end of his work would be to contribute to the cause of victory. His end as a soldier, valid as it is, is subordinated to the end of his work. A good soldier, for Aristotle, is one who willingly subordinates his own good as a worker to the end he is working for. One good is higher than the other. To take another example, a medical doctor is involved with two distinct ends, his own and the one he serves as a doctor. It would be unethical for a doctor to place his end as a worker above the end for which he works. If, for example, he performed unnecessary surgery for the purpose of enhancing his finances, he would be acting as a bad doctor. As long as he is willing to subordinate his own private interests to the health interests of his patients, he is behaving as he should as a good doctor. He behaves unethically when he inverts the hierarchy and uses his medical skills not to help patients but to gain certain personal satisfactions. Just as the very *meaning* of a soldier or a doctor is to serve the end of the work they are trained to perform, the meaning of a person is to act in a similarly self-effacing and generous way. The meaning of sex cannot be simply sex itself. Its meaning has a transcendent implication (or trans-conjugal) and involves a certain openness to new life. Contraception inverts this hierarchy so that married partners do not subordinate sexual intercourse to its higher aspirations, but subordinate the end of the work (openness or respect for new life) to the end of the workers (the partners themselves). Contracepting couples, therefore, are opposing the natural direction that the generosity of their beings as persons inclines them. They are, so to speak, at odds with themselves.

Mother Teresa, in her speech before President and Mrs. Clinton at the 1994 National Prayer Breakfast, summed up the inverted hierarchy of values that contraception represents in the following words:

> The way to plan the family is Natural Family Planning, not contraception. In destroying the power of giving life, through contraception, a husband or wife is doing something to self. This turns the attention to self and so destroys the gift of love in him or her. In loving, the husband and wife must turn the attention to each other. Once that living love is destroyed by contraception, abortion follows very easily.

The Hasidic Jewish personalist, Martin Buber, underscores the importance of a moral hierarchy in his classic work, *I-Thou*. Opposing the singularity of Descartes, Buber proposed that the two word-combinations: "I-It" and "I-Thou" are primary. And the former must be subordinated to the latter, for, as Buber explains, "without *It* man cannot live. But he who lives with *It* alone is not a man."[11]

At the heart of the person is a law of superabundance. "Life is to give," as Victor Hugo reminds us in *Les Miserables*. "Every man and every woman fully realizes himself or herself through the sincere gift of self," adds John Paul II. The most authentic meaning, in life, therefore, is to be a gift which is fully realized in the giving of oneself. In making oneself a gift for others, a person realizes his highest aim and call. Marriage offers an excellent opportunity for two persons — husband and wife — to give themselves unreservedly to each other.

Life is short, and it may be sobering to consider that in the last analysis, giving is far more realistic than taking. We cannot take with us what we have taken from life, but we can leave behind what we have given. We may envy people who are wealthy, but we admire those who are generous. We should like to think that in our own lives we were generous rather than possessive.

Because we often think in materialistic terms, however, we tend to think that to give is to become less, and to give generously is to risk becoming impoverished. The maxim that "It is better to give than to receive," does not ring true in the minds of chartered accountants.

Greed is the natural enemy of generosity. But it is important to realize that we cannot add anything to our own being through acquisition. In fact, the accumulation of things can conceal our true being from us. As many philosophers have pointed out, we must learn that the order of *having* must be subordinated to that of *being* if we are to live authentic lives. And if the law of our being is to give, we work against our own good when we fail to heed this truth.

Plato said that because God created out of pure generosity, he was incapable of envy.

We waste a lot of time envying others, whereas, in being generous we are imitating God. Another way of expressing this is to say that by being generous, we dispose ourselves to receive the bounty of a generous God who enriches us far beyond what material goods could possibly do. We should not want to contracept *ourselves* from the life that flows from God's superabundance.

Endnotes

[1] Jacques Maritain, *Existence and the Existent* (Garden City, NY: Doubleday, 1948), p. 89.

[2] Pope John Paul II, *Veritatis Splendor*, sec. 49.

[3] John F. Whitaker, M. D., "Personal Marriage Contract," *Woman's Day*, Aug. 7, 1978.

[4] Gore Vidal, "Gore Vidal: Beyond Politics and Gender," *Viva*, Nov. 1973, p. 135.

[5] Paul Vitz, "Empirical Science and Personhood," A. Moraczewski *et al.* (eds.), *Technological Powers and the Person* (St. Louis, MO: The Pope John Center, 1983), p. 207.

[6] "*Mutter, Mutter, lass uns nach Hause!/Die Tür ist verriegelt, wir finden nicht ein.* Sherrill Hahn Pantle, *Die Frau ohne Schatten* by Hugo von Hofmannsthal and Richard Strauss (Bern, Switzerland: Peter Lang, 1978), p. 48.

[7] Wanda Poltawska, "The Effect of a Contraceptive Attitude on Marriage," *International Review of Natural Family Planning*, Vol. IV, No. 3, Fall 1980, p. 205.

[8] Dr. Anne Terruwe, in *ibid.*, p. 204.

[9] Ralph McInerny, "Children: The Crown of Spousal Love," *Social Justice Review*, Nov.-Dec. 1986, p. 202.

[10] Gilbert Keith Chesterton, *G. K.'s Weekly*, Jan. 29, 1927.

[11] Martin Buber, *I-Thou* (New York, NY: Scribner's Sons, 1958), p. 34.

Contraception and Virtue

According to a commonplace expression, which is a very profound one, *man must become who he is*. Man is a *person*. He is not an extension of his environment. It is not his destiny to be socially conditioned or completely politicized. Nor is he meant to be a mere child of his times, an unthinking tool of the *Zeitgeist*. He is a person who, because he is incomplete, must complete himself through intelligence and love, through cultivating virtues and performing good deeds.

The personalist philosopher Jean Mouroux addresses this paradox when he states that "The person is a reality given and a reality still to be achieved."[1] Another personalist philosopher, Emmanual Mounier, makes the same point in declaring that "The personal is the mode of existence proper to man. Nevertheless, it has ceaselessly to be obtained."[2]

We cannot "achieve" or "attain" our fulfillment as persons without virtue. This is simply a matter of being realistic. Yet our contemporary society shows far more affection for virtual reality than it does for virtuous reality. T. S. Eliot has remarked that contemporary man is so terrified of reality that he seeks to escape from it "by dreaming of systems so perfect that no one will need to be good."[3] Aldous Huxley made reference to the world's heroic attempt to replace virtue with the wonders wrought by chemistry, in his dystopian nightmare, *Brave New World*. "Anybody can be virtuous now," he wrote. "You can carry at least half your morality about in a bottle. Christianity without tears — that's what *soma* is."[4]

To obtain "virtue in a bottle" seems far more attractive, in our Age of Convenience, than struggling to attain virtue and become an authentic person. As we exchange personal virtue for impersonal technology, we come to believe that using contraception is a virtuous act, namely the virtue of *responsibility*. Once contraception is in place, we believe that we can live virtuously as we pass from "freedom of choice" to "unbinding commitments" to "unwanted pregnancies" to "abortion on demand" to "no fault divorce." We do not stop to realize that what we took to be a comprehensive form of "sexual freedom" was actually a form of "sexual suicide." Thus, a pastor distributes condoms during a church service instead of communion;[5] a priest stands on a highway and tosses condoms at college students on their way to Ft. Lauderdale; mothers in Australia put birth control pills in the morning tea of daughters as young as twelve years old; a mother of two boasts, "I've had three abortions. Thank God I had the freedom to choose;"[6] and the vice-president of the United States blithely announces that contraception will curtail "unwanted pregnancies and abortions."[7] In response to contemporary society's collective flight from virtue, Dr. Laura Schlessinger has responded in a book with the Jeremiac title, *How Could You Do That?! The Abdication of Character, Courage, and Conscience.*[8]

Mahatma Gandhi warned the world about the dangers of relinquishing virtue for technology. He was particularly concerned about the adoption of contraception and the abdication of chastity. In a statement that brims with personalistic values, he once stated:

> I suggest that it is cowardly to refuse to face the consequences of one's acts. Persons who use contraceptives will never learn the value of self-restraint. They will not need it. Self-indulgence with contraceptives may prevent the coming of children but will sap the vitality of both men and women, perhaps more of men than of women.[9]

Such words, however, tend to fall on deaf ears as the Age of Mass-Man becomes more deeply entrenched.

The Emergence of Mass-Man

In 1930, the Spanish existentialist, José Ortega Gasset, wrote a rather provocative book called *The Revolt of the Masses* in which he distinguished two classes of men: "those who made great demands on themselves, piling up difficulties and duties; and those who demand nothing special of themselves, but for whom to live is to be every moment what they already are, without imposing on themselves any effort towards perfection; mere buoys that float on the waves."[10] The great danger Ortega alluded to at this time was the emergence and domination in society of this latter type, mass-man, who was producing a grotesque inversion of the social order through what Ortega termed the "sovereignty of the unqualified." The masses, according to Ortega, were beginning to usurp the leadership of better qualified, more responsible individuals. As a result of this refusal to improve himself as a person, mass-man was becoming more and more alienated from his better self. "Lord of all things," Ortega wrote, "he is not lord of himself. . . . Hence the strange combination of a sense of power and a sense of insecurity which has taken up its abode in the soul of modern man."

The distinction Ortega makes between the two classes of men ultimately plays itslf out on the social stage as a clash between two antithetic tendencies: civilization and barbarism. On the one hand, civilization affirms individual life, noble standards, justice and reason, while barbarism, on the other hand, in Ortega's words, "crushes beneath it everything that is excellent, individual, qualified, and select."[11]

Sixty-five years later, in 1995, Pope John Paul II produced *Evangelium Vitae* which, in effect, corroborated the main outline of Ortega's thesis. The Holy Father distinguished between a culture of death and a culture of life. He criticized the widespread and exclusive preoccupation with man's material well-being to the neglect of the more profound dimensions of human existence — the personal, interpersonal, spiritual, and religious. He pointed out that in this context of "practical materialism," suffering, which is not only an inescapable burden of human existence but also a factor in personal growth, is "censored," deemed useless, and regarded, even, as an evil that must always and in every way be avoided. For both Ortega and John Paul, mass-man was producing a culture of death largely because he rejected difficulty and suffering as indispensable factors in the equation of human, and consequently, cultural improvement.

The Pope also pointed out that in the present highly restricted atmosphere of materialism and consumerism, sexuality, too, has become depersonalized and exploited, "from being the sign, place and language of love, that is, of the gift of self and acceptance of another, in all the other's richness as a person, it increasingly becomes the occasion and instrument for self-assertion and the selfish satisfaction of personal desires and instinct."[12] He identified the use of contraception and abortion as evil acts, the former being a sin against *chastity*, the latter against *justice*, a direct violation of the commandment "You shall not kill."[13]

In the sixty-five years that separated *The Revolt of the Masses* from *Evangelium Vitae*, innumerable social critics have written about the rise of mass-man and its accompanying culture of death. Psychoanalytic humanist Erich Fromm has written extensively on the subject, reiterating that "there is no life of 'the masses'."[14] Perhaps no one has expressed modern man's proclivities to cultural annihilation more strikingly than American literary critic, Leslie Fiedler:

. . .it's difficult to avoid the conclusion that Western man has decided to abolish himself, creating his own boredom out of his
own affluence, his own vulnerability out of his own strength, his
own impotence out of his own erotomania, himself blowing the
trumpet that brings the walls of his own city tumbling down.
Having convinced himself that he is too numerous, he labours
with pill and scalpel and syringe to make himself fewer, thereby
delivering himself the sooner into the hands of his enemies. At
last, having educated himself into imbecility and polluted and
drugged himself into stupefaction, he keels over, a weary, bat-
tered old brontosaurus, and becomes extinct.[15]

In order to conform to the masses, mass-man has had to reject his
unique, personal destiny. At the same time, he has had to reject those
specific character traits which would have enabled him to achieve
that destiny. In other words, mass-man has rejected the moral virtue
needed in order to make the transformation from an undifferentiated
member of mass culture to an authentic and unique person. Nowhere is this rejection more evident than in the area of human sexuality. Chastity, the virtue that binds sexuality to reason and order, is
routinely dismissed as either unrealistic, impractical, or unnatural.
As Anatole France has cynically remarked, "Of all sexual aberra-
tions, chastity is the strangest."

The mind of the masses is nowhere more demonstrably bankrupt
than in matters of sexuality. It believes that the procreative potential
of sexual intercourse can be nullified by a contraceptive, and its capacity to transmit disease thwarted by a condom. It believes that the
lust of a sexual aggressor can be effectively tamed by the utterance of
a verbal signal. Thus, the Pill is supposed to take away the fear of
pregnancy, the condom is presumed to ensure that sex will be "safe",
and the word "No" will allegedly transform a sexual predator on the
spot into a respectful and law abiding citizen. Virtue is assumed to
be unnecessary as long as one is equipped with the approved arsenal
of slogans and technological armanentaria.

Our Materialistic World

In the interest of publicizing National Condom Week in England,
a safe-sex poster depicted Pope John Paul II wearing a hardhat. The
accompanying message read: "Eleventh Commandment: Thou Shalt
Always Wear a Condom." Britain's advertising watchdog, The Advertising Standards Authority, condemned the poster after receiving
1,187 complaints from the British Safety Council. The Council
spokesperson, however, defended the ad: "We chose this particular

image to emphasize the fact that the Catholic stance on contraception is incompatible with the concept of safe sex."[16] This gratuitous reduction of the Church's spacious teaching on human sexuality to its ban of contraception illustrates not only inexcusable ignorance, but a flat refusal to acknowledge the facts or engage in the most elementary form of thinking on the subject. The Church is not content with sex being safe; she wants it to be virtuous. She is not satisfied with hygienic robots; she wants authentic persons. But a spiritually bankrupt secular mind is riveted to a single fear — that sex can spread disease.

A poster can hardly begin to do justice to the mysteries and complexities of human sexuality. It is far more likely to exploit the unwary reader through misinformation and misunderstanding. The unhappy truth of the matter is that the sexual appetite, more than any other appetite, is most susceptible to manipulation and mis-direction. Moreover, nothing is more perilous, either to the individual or to society, than unvirtuous or disordered sex. The British social anthropologist J. D. Unwin studied the births and deaths of eighty civilizations, and concluded that no society which does not direct its sexual energies to the good of marriage and the family can survive for more than one generation.

Human sexuality is, by nature, ordinated to express love and to initiate life. But in a reductively materialistic society which demeans the spiritual verities that human sexuality introduces, sex is re-defined in specifically materialistic terms, although its spiritual essence is not completely overshadowed. Malcolm Muggeridge captured the spirit of this re-definition most aptly when he described it as the "mysticism of materialism." Human beings are inescapably spiritual. Even the most crass materialist has some sense of sex's spiritual dimension. Unfortunately, it is often treated as the only entrance into a world of spiritual values. Hence the paradox of mass-man: although he does not respect sex enough, he nonetheless expects too much from it. Or, as G. K. Chesterton once remarked, the man who is knocking on the door of a brothel, even if he does not realize it, is really looking for God.

There is a prevailing sense, even among the masses, that sex is wildly and dangerously out of control. The arch-materialists, themselves, are not at peace with their own materialism. Yet, the only cure they can imagine is more technology, which is to say, more of the disease. The root of the sexual problem, being spiritual, remains essentially unaffected by technological interventions.

Canada's foremost communications expert, the late Marshall McLuhan, stated in his first book, *The Mechanical Bride*, published in 1951, that the fusion of sex with technology represented one of the most peculiar features of the contemporary world. He saw a twofold root to this strange hybrid: a hungry curiosity to explore and enlarge the domain of sex by mechanical technique, and a desire to *possess* machines in a sexually gratifying way.[17] In either case, sex is wrenched from any direct association with love or life. Such an unlikely alliance, according to McLuhan, invites destruction. There is a mysterious link, he warned, between sex, technology, and death.[18]

A cartoon in the *New Yorker* illustrates this same fusion of sex with technology. A salesgirl, trying to sell a certain brand of perfume to a young female customer, recommends it by remarking: "It smells like a new sports-car." Erich Fromm found in this vignette an accurate image of *Homo mechanicus* who is more interested in manipulating machines than in enjoying life. In Fromm's view, the man who becomes indifferent to life and enthralled by the mechanical is "eventually attracted by death and total destruction."[19]

The distinguished urban philosopher, Lewis Mumford, who spent a long and fruitful career studying and criticizing our contemporary machine-oriented society (our "megatechnic civilization") was well aware of the contemporary mechanization of sex. In his book, *The Pentagon of Power*, he cites a "Happening" staged at an American university that exquisitely symbolizes the current fusion of sex and the machine. In this "happening," a group of women build a nest, while a group of men erect a tower. Each group then destroys the other's work. The festivities end when all participants surround an automobile covered with strawberry jam and proceed to treat it as a giant ice-cream cone. The evident symbolism is the destruction (or "deconstruction") of traditional sex roles and an erotic involvement with the machine.[20]

Sex as Dangerous

The expression "safe sex" carries the inevitable implication that sex, in its natural mode, unwed to technology, is dangerous. Natural sex becomes, in a sense, unnatural, just as traditional sex roles also appear to be unnatural. It is said that the condom helps to insure that sex does not lead to death. This is a rather audacious prediction given the Pill's abysmal history of serving as a gateway to abortion. It should not be forgotten, however, that this reductive, mechanized view of sex is precisely what established the sex-death connection in the first place. Once sex was removed from the protective context of love and life within marriage, it became immediately vulnerable to secular exploitation. Self-indulgence with contraception does not render sex safe, any more than a bad marriage with a library of self-help books immunizes a couple against divorce. The condom is like the cigarette filter. Its presence presupposes a prior danger. Healthy lungs require not the use of a cigarette filter, but the abandonment of cigarette smoking altogether and the presence of fresh air. Safe sex, if the expression has any legitimate meaning, demands the abandonment of a promiscuous attitude toward sex. In more positive terms, it requires the acquisition of virtue. To substitute a condom for virtue is to perpetuate the practice of depersonalizing sex. Virtue must be present in sexual relationships to ensure that the person is present. And the presence of the person ensures that it is the person that is paramount in sexual relationships, not the pleasure.

Unvirtuous sex is ruinous of sex. But more significantly, it is ruinous of persons. St. Thomas Aquinas lists eight daughters of unchastity, each of which contributes, in varying degrees, to the incapacitation of the person. They are: blindness of mind, rashness, thoughtlessness, inconstancy, inordinate self-love, hatred of God, excessive love of this world, and abhorrence or despair of a future world.[21] He explains that they wreak havoc with the four acts of reason and the two-fold orientation of the will. Blindness hinders one's ability to apprehend an object rightly. Rashness interferes with counsel. Thoughtlessness opposes judgment about what is to be done. And inconstancy conflicts with reason's command about what is to be done. Inordinate self-love is contrary to the will's proper end which is God, while hatred of God flows from His forbidding acts of lust. Love of this world is inimical to the means man should will in relation to his end, while despair of a future world results from the distaste of spiritual pleasures brought on by over-indulgence in the pleasures of the flesh.

Shakespeare's *Measure for Measure* offers a dramatic and compelling image of how unchastity (or lust) can bring about personal disintegration. Angelo offers to spare the life of Isabella's brother, Claudio, if she consents to sleep with him. Claudio faces death because of sexual misconduct. When Isabella, who is a novice in a cloistered order of nuns, discusses the matter with her brother, she is horrified to discover what a despicable rake he has become as a result of his carnal misadventures. "Death is a fearful thing," says Claudio, who has little regard for his sister's chastity. "And shamed life a hateful," replies Isabella. Claudio becomes more earnest in his plea: "Sweet sister, let me live: What sin you do to save a brother's life, / Nature dispenses with the deed so far / That it becomes a virtue." Her response is most emphatic:

> O you beast!
> O faithless coward! O dishonest wretch!
> Wilt thou be made a man out of my vice?
> Is't not a kind of incest, to take life
> From thine own sister's shame?

She breaks off any further discussion by exclaiming that for Claudio, fornication was not a lapse but a life-style: "Thy sin's not accident, but a trade, / Mercy to thee would prove itself a bawd: / 'Tis best that you diest quickly."[22] Claudio's preoccupation with sex, which had become a "trade," or a cold-blooded way of life, poisoned his soul to the degree that his own sister's honor meant nothing to him. In fact, poor Claudio had lost all sense of right and wrong.

The Meaning of Chastity

The words "chastity" and "unchastity" are seldom properly understood. "Chaste is waste," and "virtue can hurt you," shibboleths of mass-man operating in a culture of death, represent the antithesis of what chastity and its opposite really mean. Chastity takes its name from the fact that reason chastises (or castigates) sexual desire which, like a child, needs curbing. Aristotle speaks of the self-indulgent child whose appetite is at variance with reason, exhibiting a "lack of chastisement."[23] The word "unchastity" in its Latin root is *incestum* which literally refers to incest. The Romans used the substantive *incestum* to signify "incest," "unchastity," or "lewdness." The record of Roman literature shows that Cicero used the adverb *inceste* to mean "sinfully" or "impurely." Virgil employed the verb *incesto* in the sense of "to defile" or to "pollute," and Horace used the adjective *incestus* in referring to a "sinful person." It could hardly be argued that Roman pagans opposed unchastity because they were puritanically disposed to sex. They understood, quite sensibly, that the sexual appetite is a powerful force that needs a virtue if it is to be yoked to reason. They may not have been faithful in practicing chastity, but they knew without doubt that chastity was a virtue and that its opposite, unchastity, was a vice.

The atheist Friedrich Nietzsche, certainly no friend of Christianity, recognized the value of chastity. In *Zarathustra*, he begins his chapter "Of Chastity" by stating: "I love the forest. It is bad to live in towns: too many of the lustful live there."[24] In the Russian culture, the word for "chastity" is *tselomudrie* which means, "the wisdom of wholeness." In the Hindu tradition, chastity is part of the virtue of *brahmachariya* , or perfect control over all the senses and organs.

The reason chastity is so decidedly unpopular today is not so much because it is too much to expect a person to harmonize his sexual appetite with reason, but because he is constantly exposed to sexually seductive stimuli. Writing in the 13th century, Aquinas remarked that that "There is not much sinning because of natural desire. . . . But the stimuli of desire which man's cunning has devised are something else, and for the sake of these sins one sins very much."[25]

Modern man must be a new Ulysses who has prepared himself in advance to deal with the seductive power of the sirens. But he must also be like Perseus who knew better than to look directly into the face of Medusa. We would be wise to emulate him by utilizing the mirror of conscious reflection. As Marshall McLuhan has stated, "Without the mirror of the mind, nobody can live a human life in the face of our present mechanized dream."[26]

Philosophy and understanding are important, perhaps even necessary, in the cultivation of any virtue, especially that of chastity. At the same time, they are insufficient. Virtue is not complete, fully virtuous, unless it is an expression of love. People may be chaste because they disdain sex, are not ready for intimacy, or are fearful of contracting a disease, or of becoming pregnant. But in the absence of love, what passes for virtuous behavior is never fully virtuous. This is why Augustine spoke of virtue as the "order of love" (*ordo amoris*). Love with virtue is deed; Love without virtue is dead.

The secular world believes that sex education requires nothing more than the dispensation of information. But it is love that binds people together sexually not the sex organs themselves. Information alone may improve technique, but of itself has nothing to do with love. Moreover, information may be used in conjunction with immoral or unreasonable ends. The essential value reason plays in virtue is to direct human actions to real goods. In this regard, reason is realistic, directing the virtuous person toward reality. The absence of chastity allows lust to take over the personality, directing it away from a world of real goods to one of fantasy. Lust, therefore, cannot be a primary passion. It is a joyless, fictitious passion because it is directed toward something that is not real. Lust replaces love, which is ontological in its significance and uniquely capable of providing personal satisfaction. Whereas love is directed to *being*, lust centers itself in nonbeing. Philosopher Joseph Pieper has expressed this idea in the following way: "Unchaste abandon and the self-surrender of the soul to the world of sensuality paralyzes the primordial powers of the moral person: the ability to perceive in silence the call of reality and to make, in the retreat of this silence, the decision appropriate to the concrete situation of concrete action."[27]

C. S. Lewis, in his most popular work, *The Screwtape Letters*, has Screwtape advise his apprentice devil, Wormwood, to "direct the desires of men to something which does not exist — making the rôle of the eye in sexuality more and more important and at the same time making its demands more and more impossible. What follows you can easily forecast!"[28]

Because lust is linked with unreality, it is not likely that one could rely on a lustful person to tell the truth. The secular world is loathe to recognize this point. While it insists that it is realistic to expect that people will be unchaste, it is equally insistent that it is realistic to expect them not to be untruthful when it comes to disclosing the state of their sexual health to their prospective sex partner. It is only too well known, needless to say, that a sexually inflamed male will often say anything if he thinks it will help him to have his way. "I love you," is now being said across the land with deadly insincerity. Or, in the words of the immortal Bard: "I do know, when the blood burns, how the prodigal soul lends the tongue vows."[29]

The acceptance of unchastity makes it difficult for people to tell the truth about sex, especially when they are aroused. The glib talk about the condom making sex safe flies in the face of the medical evidence. The *Journal of the American Medical Association* reports that 30% of previously uninfected spouses of AIDS-infected individuals seroconverted (became infected with the HIV virus) after an average of one year of using condoms with their infected partners. Other studies have reported similar results.[30]

Chastity operates on two levels. There is the specific virtue of chastity that regulates sexual desires and actions so that they are in accord with reason. Then there is chastity in the metaphorical sense which allows the mind to be united with the natural and even the Divine order of things. It gives the soul a certain transparence. "Blessed are the pure of heart, for they shall see God" (Mt. 5: 8). In this sense, Aquinas writes, "the essence of chastity consists principally in charity and the other theological virtues, whereby the human mind is united to God."

We need chastity in both senses if we are to have chastity at all. Chastity begins and ends in love. The world hungers for love, though it does not know how to find it. What it does know is the value of its information and technique. These are real and tangible; chastity is presumed not to be. Nonetheless, neither information nor technique can enrich life nor give it meaning. Love alone can achieve that. Even so, love must not be pursued apart from faith and hope. Chastity, within or prior to marriage, is not unrealistic; it is only too realistic, involving more of ourselves than we understand. And if we are sometimes discouraged, we might find comfort and encouragement in these words of C. S. Lewis:

> At present we are on the outside of the world, the wrong side of
> the door. We discern the freshness and purity of
> morning, but they do not make us fresh and pure. We cannot
> mingle with the splendors we see. But all the leaves of the
> the New Testament are rustling with the rumor that it will not al-
> ways be so. Some day, God willing, we shall get in.[31]

Endnotes

[1]Jean Mouroux, *The Meaning of Man* (New York, NY: Sheed & Ward, 1948), p. 144.

[2]Emmanuel Mounier, *Personalism* (New York, NY: Grove Press, 1952), p. xi.

[3]T. S. Eliot, "Choruses from 'the Rock'," *The Complete Poems and Plays* (New York, NY: Harcourt, Brace & World, 1952), p. 106.

[4]Aldous Huxley, *Brave New World* (New York, NY: Time, 1963), p. 208.

[5]"Pastor joins more to back 'safe sex'." *USA Today*, Feb. 6, 1987, p. 2A.

[6]"Areas Biggest Abortion Provider Has Busy Day," *St. Louis Post Dispatch*, Jan. 18, 1998.

[7]Vice-President Al Gore, *EWTN news brief*, Jan. 23, 1998.

[8]Laura Schlessinger, *How Could You Do That?! The Abdication of Character, Courage, and Conscience* (New York, NY: HarperCollins, 1996).

[9]Mahatma Gandhi, *Wisdom for all Time: Mahatma Gandhi and Pope Paul VI on Birth Regulation,* prepared by A. S. Antonisamy, (Pondicherry, India: Family Life Service Centre, 1978), p. 26.

[10]José Ortega Gasset, *The Revolt of the Masses* (New York, NY: Mentor Books, 1950), p. 10.

[11]*Ibid.,* pp. 31-2, 12.

[12]John Paul II, *Evangelium Vitae*, sec. 23.

[13]*Ibid.,* sec. 13.

[14]Erich Fromm. *The Heart of Man* (New York, NY: Harper & Row, 1971), p. 63.

[15]Leslie Fiedler, quoted in *Trousered Apes* by Duncan Williams.

[16]"Condom ads too cheeky," *The Toronto Sun*, Sept. 7, 1995, p. 43.

[17]Marshall McLuhan, *The Mechanical Bride* (Boston, MA: Beacon Press, 1967), p. 43.

[18]*Ibid.,* p. 101.

[19]Fromm, *op. cit.,* p. 65.

[20]Lewis Mumford, *The Pentagon of Power* (New York, NY: Harcourt, Brace, & Jovanovich, 1970), p. 365.

[21]Aquinas, *Summa Theologica*, II-II, 153, 5.

[22]William Shakespeare, *Measure for Measure*, III, i.

[23]Aristotle, *Ethics*, III, 12.

[24]Friedrich Nietzsche, *Thus Spake Zarathustra,* tr. By R. J. Hollingdale (Harmondsworth, Middlesex, England: Penguin Books, 1969), p. 81.

[25]Joseph Pieper, "Chastity and Unchastity," *The Four Cardinal Virtues* (New York, NY: Harcourt, Brace & World, 1965), p. 173.

[26]McLuhan, *op. cit.,* p. 97.

[27]Pieper, *op. cit.,* p. 160.

[28]C. S. Lewis, *The Screwtape Letters* (New York, NY: Time Incorporated, 1960), pp. 69-70.

[29]William Shakespeare, *Hamlet,* I, 3, 116.

[30]*Journal of American Medical Association,* Dec. 18, 1987.

[31]C. S. Lewis, *Transposition and other Addresses* (London, England: Geoffrey Bles, 1949), p. 31.

Contraception, Revolution, and Prophecy

For the multitudes who find little meaning and even less hope in their day-to-day existence, nothing short of the prospect of a revolution is required to arouse them to action. Perhaps no words have been more eagerly received by such citizens of the modern era than those clothed in the glittering rhetoric that flashed from the pages of Marx' and Engels' *Communist Manifesto*:

> Let the ruling classes tremble at a Communist revolution. The proletarians have nothing to lose but their chains. They have a world to win. Working men of all countries, unite!

The rhetoric of revolution appeals to people who are hungry for two things: sweeping improvements and their speedy implementation, if not immediate delivery. Such people are neither willing to abide the *status quo* or to wait much longer for release from their unhappy burdens. The words "liberation" and "now" become shibboleths for promoting the revolution and are on the lips of everyone who espouses its cause.

Revolution is opposed to *devolution*; it is progressive, rather than regressive. It is also opposed to *evolution* inasmuch as it evolves quickly rather than slowly. Revolution, therefore, has two essential features: one that represents a major improvement of some kind, the other involving an interval of time that is as brief as possible. In sum, a social revolution is a form of progress that plays on people's dissatisfaction with their lives and an impatience about their improvement.

Two Revolutions

In the decade of the 1960's, two important revolutions intertwined: the Sexual and Contraceptive Revolutions. The Sexual Revolution promised a more healthy, less inhibited sexual life-style, and the Contraceptive Revolution made possible, at least theoretically, its immediate delivery. Together, this revolutionary tandem promised an attractive array of human improvements: less sexual frustration, better marriages, fewer divorces, better child spacing, fewer unwanted pregnancies, a higher percentage of wanted babies, fewer abortions, and an easing of the population crisis. It preached an only

97

too familiar line of rhetoric to its potential beneficiaries: "Let the authoritarians tremble at a Sexual Revolution. The masses have nothing to lose but their inhibitions. They have a world of sexual fulfillment to win. Men and women everywhere, unite!"

The Catholic Church's endorsement of the rhythm method had not been favorably received by the world at large. The "rhythm" or "calendar" method was mockingly labeled as "Vatican Roulette," and it was commonly joked that people who practiced it were known as "parents." Nor was the media cordial to the rhythm method. Journalist H. L. Mencken, for example, had derisively commented that "It is now quite lawful for a Catholic woman to avoid pregnancy by a resort to mathematics, though she is still forbidden to resort to physics or chemistry." The Church's opposition to contraception, however, has always been moral, not scientific. But, even the now out-moded rhythm method presupposed specialized knowledge of physics and chemistry. The Church is most assuredly well disposed toward scientific disciplines. In fact, she draws upon the knowledge they provide in developing Natural Family Planning approaches that include such scientific paraphernalia as symptothermal detection instruments, ovulation measuring devices, and ultra-sound scanning machines. At the heart and core of systematic NFP is the scientific method — the systematic observation and recording of recurring natural events.

Society's criticisms of Church teaching on sexual matters only intensified, however, as the Sexual and Contraceptive Revolutions gathered momentum. The Church was one of the few social forces that firmly opposed the tide of this joint revolution. As a consequence, it became an easy and frequent target of criticism. To an increasing number of people, the Church appeared more backward, medieval, anti-scientific, and Puritanical, than ever before. To cite but one representative example, Dr. Albert Ellis, a popular speaker and author of some 40 books on sex, advised the Church to endorse pre-marital sex. "If it doesn't," he flatly predicted, it will "go out of business."

At this time of fierce opposition between the Church and the world, a scientist who identified himself as a devout Catholic entered the fray with the expressed hope of saving the Church from what he termed "medievalism." Dr. John Rock, a Harvard professor of gynecology, achieved national fame virtually overnight with his publication in 1963 of *The Time Has Come: A Catholic Doctor's Proposals to End the Battle over Birth Control.* In this book, Dr. Rock advised his Church to accept the Pill. A large measure of the doctor's credibility lay in the fact that he was presumed to be, in all other respects, an orthodox Catholic. Nonetheless, having noted that the Church lost its fight on birth control, he predicted it would also lose the fight on sterilization and abortion. In 1973, the year of *Roe v. Wade*, Dr. Rock stated that "given the reality of malnutrition in the world, efforts to prevent abortions were a blasphemy."[1]

When *Humanae Vitae* appeared in 1968, the world had been conditioned to reject it. In the spring of 1967, *Newsweek* published the results of an extensive survey that claimed that the percentage of American Catholics who approved contraception had greatly increased, to 73%. The survey also reported that more Catholics had come to accept abortion, divorce, and optional celibacy for priests.[2]

Historian James Hitchcock draws the conclusion that "The rejection of *Humanae Vitae* was hardly spontaneous. It was preceded by at least five years when the most influential segments of the media, secular and Catholic, propagandized intensely for a change in the official teaching. Although there was much talk of 'dialogue' and 'pluralism', in fact the discussion was remarkably one-sided." Hitchcock also pointed out that the so-called "population crisis" was, in countless articles and radio and television broadcasts, presented as a moral imperative that could neither be denied nor compromised.[3]

Moral Growth

Revolutions may be intellectual, political, or technological; they are rarely, if ever, moral. Proponents of the Sexual-Contraceptive Revolution severely misjudged it as a moral phenomenon when, in reality, it was largely technological. Moral improvements are arduous and slow. When they occur, they usually require a long period of time, that is to say, *they evolve.*

Placing sex within a revolutionary framework dooms it from the start. Sex is not something to be liberated; rather, it is the human being who stands in need of liberation. But even here, the liberation must be *evolutionary*, not revolutionary.

The salient fact that the Sexual-Contraceptive Revolution is characterized by an obsession with sex is a clear indication that sex has not been properly integrated into the whole of human existence. Sex had been separated rather than liberated: separated from love, marriage, life, intimacy, and commitment. It has been thereby isolated. In this unnatural state it appears larger than life and as such appears to be an object of disproportionate importance and obsessive interest.

When a person is healthy, his attention is not concentrated on any particular part of his body. But if he has a splitting headache, he can think of little else. Kurt Goldstein comments in his work *Human*

Nature in the Light of Psychopathology that "the hedonistic tendency originates in the abnormal isolation of one attribute of human nature. In consequence [the hedonist] is incapable of experiencing the positive character of joy." People have "sex on the brain," as Malcolm Muggeridge has noted, and "that's an unhealthy place for it to be."

Moral growth is slow because there are so many factors to integrate. Information needs to be integrated into knowledge, knowledge has to be tempered by wisdom, action needs to be modified by experience. Knowledge needs love, love needs virtue, virtue needs experience, experience needs time. Family members understand well that "home wasn't built in a day." In his work, *Freedom in the Modern World*, Catholic philosopher Jacques Maritain underscores how a moral change in the heart is indispensable for any external change that is worth striving for:

> To wish to change the face of the earth without first changing one's heart (which no man can do of his own strength) is to undertake a work that is purely destructive. Perhaps indeed if omnipotent love did truly transform our hearts, the exterior work of reform would already be half done.

Moral *evolutions* and technological *revolutions* are essentially at odds with each other because of the contradictory ways in which they evaluate time. The former cherishes time, the latter contemns it. When the German poet Hölderlein stated that "the unmindful God abhors untimely growth," he was alluding to the fact that it is natural for human growth to be slow and unhurried. Feeding rapid growth fertilizer to weeds causes them to grow out of their roots and perish. A similar calamity awaits the human being who tries to grow at a faster pace than nature will allow. Organic growth demands that all the parts evolve together in balance. The isolation and obsession with one part can be ruinous to the good of the whole.

Jonathan Livingston Seagull wants to fly at instantaneous speed. This fictional character is emblematic of contemporary society's excessive preoccupation with speed. People who are impatient in their quest for pleasure often choose the quick fix: drugs, alcohol, pornography. But everything organic, especially the organic quality of moral values, takes time. The aphorism "haste makes waste" is particularly true when a technological short-cut substitutes for moral development.

The Sexual Revolution failed because it demanded that sex be removed from its proper context of organic wholeness and enjoyed independently of any natural association with complementary moral values. The Contraceptive Revolution failed because technological control was used in the place of personal control (self-control) which immediately led to an erosion of personal integrity.

The Failed Revolution

As the Revolution advanced, more and more people were witness to its negative direction. Dr. Robert Kistner, a gynecological surgeon who had worked with doctors John Rock and Gregory Pincus in developing the Pill, said, in 1977: "I felt the Pill would not lead to promiscuity. But I have changed my mind. I think it probably has and so has the IUD."

Given the wave of sexually transmitted diseases the Revolution brought about, even its most ardent promoters had to recognize problems. *Rolling Stone* magazine speculated that "some wrathful deity is exacting revenge for our decade-long orgy" as a way of possibly accounting for the epidemic of venereal disease and other sexual miseries.[4] In that same year, *Time* magazine reported that an estimated ten million Americans now had infectious, incurable herpes. Sex as a consumer item was not working, though this unhappy consequence surprised a number of people, for, as *Time* stated: ". . .in the age of the Pill, Penthouse Pets, and porn-movie cassettes, the revolution looked so sturdily permanent that sex seemed to subside into a simple consumer item."[5]

In 1971, zero-populationist Ellen Peck stated in her best-selling book, *The Baby Trap*, that the Pill should be regarded as natural and just a casual "part of a girl's totebag equipment or make-up paraphernalia." But by 1984, liberationist Germaine Greer, after a long and torturous Odyssey, came to agree that "Most of the pleasure in the world is still provided by children and not by genital dabbling."[6]

In a 1987 article entitled, "Whatever happened to the Contraceptive Revolution?", Richard Lincoln and Lisa Kaeser of the contraception-promoting Alan Guttmacher Institute in New York, stated:

> Indeed, if, in the 1960's we witnessed a contraceptive revolution, then in the 1980's we are seeing the failure of that revolution and the reversal of so many of its hard-won gains.[7]

The Revolution was yielding disappointing results, even on a demographic scale, to the alarm of some population-watchers. Demographer Pierre Chenu writes:

> Since 1964 — the take-off point for most European countries — we have arrived at a process of reproductive collapse never before seen in history. From a gradual death we are moving to an

instantaneous death: Germany is dead; its situation is non-reversible (1.2 children per German woman, while an average of 2.1 children per woman is necessary to replace a generation). How is this implosion, this destruction explained? The most blame apparently can be assigned to the contraceptive revolution which started in 1960.[8]

In Catholic circles, Lawrence Cardinal Shehan of Baltimore took stock of the Revolution's progress five years after the release of *Humanae Vitae* and had the following appraisal:

Contraception had failed to produce any of the advantages its advocates foretold with so much confidence: the stability of the family; the fall of the divorce rate; the decline of juvenile delinquency; the lessening of the problems of poverty; etc. It can be said without fear of contradiction that during the time the contraception movement had flourished, most, if not all, of these problems have increased.[9]

The Cardinal's evaluation appears as a confirmation of the predictions Pope Paul VI made in his Encyclical which applied to those who separated the procreative aspect of sex from its unitive purpose. How easy it would be, the Pope warned those who violated this law by which the unitive and procreative ends of sex are bound together, to weaken marriage, justify infidelity, bring about a lessening of respect husbands would have for their wives, contribute to a general moral decline, and leave the young without proper and adequate sexual guidance.[10]

In the anthology that scholar Janet Smith edited, *Why Humanae Vitae Was Right*, published 25 years after *Humanae Vitae*, Professor Smith characterized the moral devastation that the sexual revolution brought about as a "sexual holocaust." "One of the prophecies made in *Humanae Vitae*," she wrote, "was that the widespread use of contraception would lead to a 'general decline in morality'. Who can deny that such has happened, especially in the sexual realm?"[11] She enumerated a litany of tribulations including the dramatic rise in the incidence of premarital sexual activity, out-of-wedlock marriage, abortions, divorces, sexually transmitted diseases, and a virtual tidal wave of pornography. "It would be unthinkable," she adds, "not to count contraception among the contributing factors."[12]

The Contraceptive Revolution failed not only because of moral reasons, but for technical and physiological reasons as well. In the United States, of 40,000 Pill users who went through a screening test, only 500 were using the Pill five years later. The main reason for this exceedingly high discontinuation rate (98.75% or 79 in 80) is the Pill's adverse side-effects, which are many and often serious. Similarly, in

Great Britain, a Royal College of General Practitioners' study reported that of 6,324 women on the Pill, only 799 (12.6%) were still taking it at the end of two years.[13] Other forms of contraceptives vary in their effectiveness in preventing pregnancy. Dr. Christopher Tietze, the late bio-statistician for Planned Parenthood, recommended the use of barrier methods of contraception backed up by abortion as the safest regimen of fertility regulation at any age.

Because contraception had not been fully reliable from a technical standpoint, and because of its undesirable side-effects, more and more people throughout the world are turning to sterilization and abortion as a way of controlling procreation. Some 40 to 60 million induced abortions take place every year and about 130 million men and women worldwide have been sterilized. Today, abortion and sterilization are the two most widely used methods of family planning. At the same time, it becomes increasingly clear that the real choice concerning birth regulation is not between contraception and sterilization or abortion, but between Natural Family Planning and sterilization or abortion.

In his article entitled, "Contraception — The Revolution that Failed," Peter Brady states:

> The prevalence of abortion, the urgent calls for the introduction of the abortifacient pill, RU 486, and the widespread recourse to permanent sterilization are the most convincing evidence of the fact that the contraceptive revolution which Dr. Rock helped to initiate in the 1960's had not fulfilled its promise. Quite simply, it has failed.[14]

The Fulfilled Prophecy

It was another Rock, the Rock of Peter, whose predictions — prophecies, rather — have been fulfilled. In the words of Bernard Nathanson, who once presided over 70,000 abortions, and is now a leading spokesman for the pro-life movement:

> To me, the encyclical *Humanae Vitae* by Pope Paul VI is curiously and eerily prophetic, with its emphasis on the two meanings of the conjugal act, the unitive and the procreative; its absolute proscription of the act of abortion; its prediction of the grave consequences of the methods for artificial birth control, such as infidelity and a general decline in morality; and its warning that such technology is a dangerous weapon when placed in the hands of public authorities who take no heed of moral exigencies.[15]

Pope Paul VI's warning to the governments of the world reads as follows:

> And then [let reasonable individuals] also carefully consider that a dangerous power will be put into the hands of rulers who care

little about the moral law. Would anyone blame those in the highest offices of the state for employing a solution [contraception] considered morally permissible for spouses seeking to solve a family difficulty, when they strive to solve certain difficulties affecting the whole nation? Who will prevent public authorities from favoring what they believe to be the most effective contraceptive methods and from mandating that everyone must use them, whenever they consider it necessary?[16]

The Pope makes two very important points in this passage. The first accords with the Church's principle of subsidiarity. Because the family is not only a small unit of society, but one that should be bound together by lines of intimate love, it is the family rather than society in general that assumes the critical task of imparting moral values to its children. But if parents are delinquent in grasping the importance of integrating the unitive and procreative ends of sex and pass on to their own children a contraceptive philosophy, can one expect the government, whose ties with children are far more loose and bureaucratic, to do any better? Can one expect the government to be better at parenting and at imparting moral values to children than parents themselves? Inevitably, morally delinquent parents will open the door for even more delinquent governing officials.

The second point refers to the government's inclination to exercise coercion to control people's actions and the consequences of these actions when the people themselves are unable to control them. Abdicating the freedom to live morally is a *carte blanche* invitation for the government to employ force in controlling human behavior. Evidence for such coercion is increasingly apparent. Numerous legislative bills have been introduced in the United States either mandating the use of the long-term contraceptive, Norplant, by women convicted of certain crimes or for providing an incentive for its use by women who are poor. One governor has proposed that his State offer free Norplant inserts to women on welfare and free vasectomies to men leaving prison. He also suggests that such forms of birth control be made mandatory in some cases. A former presidential candidate proposed that poor mothers be paid $100 per year as an incentive to use Norplant. Norplant inserts are offered free of charge at a Baltimore public high school to teenage mothers without parental knowledge or consent. The program has drawn praise from the *New York Times* and is likely to serve as a model for other schools.

The loss of control of sex leads to eroticism that prompts the State to impose order by force. Thus eroticism leads to totalitarianism. This latter point has been eloquently articulated by the Irish prelate, Cardinal Cahal Daly:

[The birth control mentality] means the abandonment of self-control over sexual urges; it implicitly authorizes sexual promiscuity. Society makes it unnaturally difficult for people, particularly young people, to be continent; and then offers a remedy, contraceptives, which merely increases the incontinence. Promiscuity is the logic of birth control; but to have promiscuity with impunity there must also be abortion and infanticide, sterilization and euthanasia. The logical contraceptionists must insist if these cannot be generalized by persuasion, they must by imposed by law. It has long been recognized that there is a connection between eroticism and totalitarianism.[17]

The merging of the failed Contraceptive Revolution and the fulfilled prophecy of Pope Paul VI has significance that goes far beyond that of an interesting, perhaps curious observation. It provides a near ideal opportunity for explaining why the Revolution failed and for illuminating an understanding of human sexuality that is healthy, personal, integrated, and realistic. In addition, it provides an opportunity for motivating people to succeed where this technological revolution failed, by inspiring a plan of moral evolution that requires time, demands love, and promises to make things more and not less difficult.

The primal divorce from which emerged many other divorces is that between the unitive and procreative. But this split, which many thought to be insignificant and without consequence, is really a separation between man and God, and the usurpation by man of the throne of God. Dietrich von Hildebrand saw the matter in these terms, and his words apply to abortion and euthanasia as well as to contraception:

We can now see more clearly the difference between natural and artificial birth control. The sinfulness of artificial birth control is rooted in the arrogation of the right to separate the actualized love union in marriage from a possible conception, to sever the wonderful, deeply mysterious connection instituted by God. This mystery is approached in an irreverent attitude. Here we are confronted with the fundamental sin of irreverence toward God, the denial of our creaturehood, the acting as if we were our own lords. . . . It is the same sinfulness that lies in suicide or in euthanasia, in both of which we act as if we were masters of life.[18]

The new moral evolution will succeed by means of renewed efforts at integrating fundamental polarities: Man and God, love and life, man and woman, Church and Christ, progress and principles, time and eternity. These integrations may be difficult, even painful; but they are redeeming. As the poet Emerson has remarked, "God offers to every mind its choice between truth and repose."

In the final paragraph of *Humanae Vitae*, Pope Paul VI alludes to one final pair of opposites that requires integration, namely, education and charity. Education is needed to commence an understanding of the laws inscribed in nature. Charity is needed to begin putting these laws into practice. That the Pope places education first is not without significance.

The world has been tireless in its attempt to put love ahead of education as if human beings could lovingly express sexuality without first serving an apprenticeship in studying its nature and structure. Separated from structure (or *relationship* from *being*), however, implies that the nature of sex is the very factor that sex must be liberated from. But charity is not blind, and best expresses itself when it knows what it is doing. The primacy of the speculative does not replace love; it gives it a realistic context so that love is true charity and not mere sentiment. The failure of the Revolution should occasion a rebirth of enthusiasm for the primacy of education. The fulfillment of the Pope's prophecy should bring to mind Christ's unwavering and protective love for His Church, and therefore urge His people to anchor their love in learning and crown their learning with love.

Endnotes

[1]*Boston Globe Sunday Magazine*, reprinted in the *St. Louis Post-Dispatch*, Aug. 20, 1973, p. 2B

[2]*Newsweek*, March 20, 1967.

[3]James Hitchcock, "The American Press and Birth Control: Preparing the Ground for Dissent," *Homiletic & Pastoral Review*, July 1980, p. 11.

[4]*Rolling Stone Magazine*, March 4, 1982.

[5]*Time*, Aug. 2, 1982.

[6]*Maclean's*, April 19, 1984.

[7]Richard Lincoln and Lisa Kaeser, "Whatever happened to the Contraceptive Revolution?," *International Family Planning Perspectives*, Dec. 1987, p. 141.

[8]Cited by Thierry Dejond, S.J. in *Contraception: the world, the flesh and the materialistic view of man* (Gaithersburg, MD: Human Life International, 1992), pp. 3-4

[9]*Homiletic & Pastoral Review*, Nov./Dec. 1973.

[10]Paul VI, *Humanae Vitae*, sec. 17.

[11]Janet Smith (ed.) *Why Humanae Vitae Was Right: A Reader* (San Francisco, CA: Ignatius Press, 1993), p. 11.

[12]*Ibid.*, p. 521.

[13]Dr. Ellen Grant, *Sexual Chemistry: Hormones, The Pill and HRT* (London, ENgland: Reed Consumer Books Ltd., 1994), p. 174.

[14]Peter Brady, "Contraception — The Revolution that Failed," *Linacre*, Feb. 1990.

[15]Bernard Nathanson, "Keynote Address, *Humanae Vitae*: Going 'Back to the Future'." Russell E. Smith (ed.), *Trust the Truth* (Braintree, MA: Pope John Center, 1991), p. 1.

[16]*Humanae Vitae*, sec. 13.

[17]*Fellowship of Catholic Scholars Newsletter*, March 1993, p. 11.

[18]Dietrich von Hildebrand, *Love, Marriage and the Catholic Conscience*, tr. by Damian Fedoryka and John Crosby (Manchester, NH: Sophia Institute Press, 1998), pp. 45-46.

Contraception and Catholic Teaching

In the first question of his *Summa Theologica*, Saint Thomas Aquinas explains why we need more than mere philosophy in order to find our way in life and attain salvation. "The truth about God," he writes, "such as reason could discover, would be known only by a few, and that after a long time, and with the admixture of many errors."[1]

For the same reasons, we need to have at our disposal not only the truth about God as revealed by Holy Scripture, but also the truths about God and man that are taught by the Catholic Church as her received Magisterium. As Aquinas writes elsewhere, "If the only way open to us for the knowledge of God were solely that of reason, the human race would remain in the blackest of ignorance."[2]

Professor Janet E. Smith, who is among the world's foremost researchers, writers, and lecturers on the Church's teaching concerning contraception, provides a good illustration of how easy it is for people to adjust to the darkness of their own ignorance. When Dr. Smith, who teaches philosophy at the University of Dallas, in Irving, Texas, introduces the topic of contraception to her students, the overwhelming majority indicate their disagreement with Church teaching. But when she asks them if they are familiar with the reasons the Church offers in condemning contraception, she finds few, if any, who are. When she asks them whether they think they are entitled to an opinion, let alone a fair opinion, on a subject about which they have read and thought little or nothing, she finds that they begin to look a bit shame-faced.[3]

On a more positive note, she finds that when students have a chance to read and discuss the encyclical *Humanae Vitae*, a good number of them not only appreciate the Church's wisdom on the subject of contraception, but accept it in a way that transforms their lives.

Pressures to conform to the world's way of viewing contraception come from many sources and are very powerful. Pope Paul VI made note of this in *Humanae Vitae*, the Church's most definitive denunciation of contraception. "It is not surprising," he wrote, "the Church finds herself a *sign of contradiction* — just as her Founder. But this is no reason for the Church to abandon the duty entrusted to her of preaching the whole moral law and the law of God."

Marriage and the World

Secular society, concerned as it is with worldly things, is not well disposed to hear the message of *Humanae Vitae*. Wealthy nations are concerned about maintaining or improving their comfortable standard of living. In order to protect this interest, they sell programs to undeveloped countries of population control that heavily emphasize the use of contraception. These countries often have little choice but to accept these programs, especially when their acceptance is the very condition upon which more legitimate forms of government aid are granted.

The United Nation's conferences on the family and on women, held in Cairo in 1994 and in Beijing in 1995, epitomize the secular imperative that a low fertility rate achieved through government-enforced contraception is the key to progress, both for women as individuals as well as for nations as a whole. This dubious association of progress with the employment of contraception on a massive scale makes it appear that the cause of some of the world's most serious problems is female fertility. As one astute observer has remarked in criticizing the UN's prevailing contraceptive strategy: "All the UN approaches to women are subsumed by the driving need to control and curtail their fertility."[4]

Material concerns are often a decisive factor for many married couples. Children are expensive and require a considerable investment in time, care, and attention. It is easy to regard them as incompatible with a life-style of material comfort. Contraception appears to be a simple and effective way for such couples to limit their family without compromising their life-style.

People who reject the Church's teaching on contraception, by and large, do so not because they understand and disagree with it, but largely because their commitment to a certain life-style prevents them from giving the Church a fair hearing. Nonetheless, they do offer "reasons" for dismissing Church teaching. They often accuse the Church of being excessively idealistic, or simply unrealistic, or out of step with the modern world, or lacking compassion for the economic and psychological hardships couples must undergo in having and raising children.

The Church teaching concerning contraception is not primarily negative, but based on a most positive understanding of marriage, sexuality, and God. Marriage, in the truest sense, is not an arbitrary arrangement, but an institution established by Christ (Mt. 19: 3 ff.; Mk. 10: 2 ff.) Marriage, therefore, is divinely instituted. This lofty, exalted understanding of marriage is nowhere better realized than in sexual union where the human act of husband and wife comes into intimate relationship with the creative act of God. Sexual union between husband and wife takes place on holy ground, as it were, since it is the place where God's creation and the married couple's procreation of new life intersect.

It is most fitting, when in the presence of God, or in a holy place, to show appropriate signs of reverence. Just as God asked Moses to remove his shoes when he was standing in the Divine presence,[5] and just as people kneel when they come into Church, it is also appropriate for married couples not to defile the holy ground, which is their sexual union and intimacy with God, with the employment of contraceptive devices.

The essential purpose of contraception is to prevent the initiation of new life. The use of contraception, therefore, represents a choice that is essentially "contralife."[6] Moreover, since God is the Creator of new life, contraception is not only contralife but contra-God-the-creator.

The notion that husband and wife become two-in-one-flesh through sexual union implies that each presents to the other the gift of self. This is the meaning of love, to give of oneself to one's beloved. The sexual act between husband and wife, however, represents a very pure form of love since it requires the spouses to love each other unreservedly and whole-heartedly. Contraception, since it is a way of holding back by not including the procreative dimension of one's being, compromises the two-in-one-flesh unity of the marital act. The use of contraception is not compatible with the kind of pure and total gift that marriage asks of husband and wife.

Church Teaching on Contraception

Contraception negates the creative act of God. It also compromises the unity of the relationship between the marriage partners. For these two reasons, fundamentally, the Church teaches that contraception is disordered and morally wrong. It is wrong, according to the Church, because it separates the procreative and the unitive meanings of the marital act. In this way, the Church condemns contraception primarily because it violates the goods of marriage and procreation. In *Humanae Vitae* we find the following statement:

> By safeguarding both these essential aspects, the unitive and the procreative, the conjugal act preserves in its fullness the sense of true marital love and its orientation toward man's exalted vocation to parenthood.[8]

In the same document, the denunciation of contraceptives of every kind is most clear: "every action which, whether in anticipation of the conjugal act, or in its accomplishment, or in the development of its natural consequences, proposes, whether as an end or as a means, to render procreation impossible" is intrinsically evil.[9] Here, the Church is explicitly rejecting such forms of contraception as the Pill, condoms, and spermicides.

Sexual intercourse is naturally ordered to procreation. This order, like the way leaves are ordered to produce food by undergoing photosynthetic activity in the presence of sunlight, exemplifies the natural law. In the Latin text of *Humanae Vitae* (Latin is the official language of the Church), the expression *"per se destinatus"* (in itself ordered) is used to indicate the natural relationship that exists between intercourse and procreation. What Church teaching opposes is the violation of the natural ordination between intercourse and the initiation of new life that God, Himself, has established. The Church does not oblige people to have as many children as possible, or to engage in sexual intercourse every time the wife appears to be fertile. She teaches that if the married spouses do have sexual union, that they do not deliberately attempt to negate the natural order that God established between the marital act and His power to create new life. Contraception, so to speak, slams the door in the face of God and encloses the married couple in a world that is deprived of important avenues of grace and therefore to sources of supernatural help.

At the same time, the Church does not forbid married couples from enjoying conjugal love when they know that procreation is either unlikely or impossible. The Church has no objection whatsoever to married couples making love when the wife is already known to be pregnant, when the wife or husband are infertile, or when the partners themselves are infertile as a couple. As Pope Paul VI states in *Humanae Vitae*: "Marital acts do not cease being legitimate if they are foreseen to be infertile because of reasons independent of the spouses."

Similarly, the Church does not require people to pray all the time. But she does hold that whenever a person prays to God, he does so with reverence. Although we need not pray always, we are never permitted to blaspheme. This negative prohibition should not be difficult to grasp since it is readily understood in thousands of commonplace circumstances. For example, while it is not required that a husband always talk to his wife, it is required that when he does speak to her, that he should do so respectfully. A wife is not obliged to prepare all meals, but when she does prepare a meal, she should not deliberately render it indigestible.

The understanding that intercourse is naturally linked to procreation has enjoyed a long and consistent history. All Christians churches were solidly united against the use of contraception until 1930 when, at the Lambeth Conference in England, the Anglican Church allowed married couples to use contraception, but only for grave reasons.

Sigmund Freud, who had little sympathy for religion of any kind, regarded the separation of intercourse from its procreative end as a model of sexual perversity. The founder of modern psychoanalysis wrote: "...it is a characteristic common to all the perversions that in them reproduction as an aim is put aside. This is actually the criterion by which we judge whether a sexual activity is perverse — if it departs from reproduction in its aims and pursues the attainment of gratification independently.... Everything that.... serves the pursuit of gratification alone is called by the unhonored title of 'perversion' and as such is despised."[10]

Throughout her history the Catholic Church has maintained a clear, forceful, and consistent position in her teaching about the essential evil of contraception. After surveying the Church's historical teaching on contraception, Paul VI's Minority Report offered the following statement:

> One can find no period in history, no document of the Church, no theological school, scarcely one Catholic theologian, who ever denied that contraception was always seriously evil. The teaching of the Church in this matter is absolutely constant. Until the present century this teaching was peacefully possessed by all other Christians, whether Orthodox or Anglican or Protestant.[11]

On December 31, 1930, only four and one-half months after the Lambeth Conference opened the doors to contraception for the Anglican Church, Pope Pius XI issued his encyclical *Casti Connubii* ("On Chaste Wedlock") in which he reiterated the Church's long-standing opposition to contraception, while explaining that, for right reasons, it is permissible to confine conjugal acts to known periods of infertility.

In 1980, at the Synod of Bishops, representatives of national hierarchies from around the world addressed the issue of contraception. After giving the matter careful consideration, the bishops professed their agreement with *Humanae Vitae* and Vatican II's *Gaudium et Spes* on contraception. John Paul II ratified their statement and, reflecting on the significance of the matter at hand, stated:

Consideration in depth of all the aspects of these problems offers a new and stronger confirmation of the importance of the authentic teaching on birth regulation reproposed in the Second Vatican Council and in the Encyclical *Humanae Vitae*.[12]

Scholars have provided highly detailed and lengthy argumentation that the Catholic Church's teaching concerning contraception has been infallibly taught by the ordinary magisterium under the conditions articulated by Vatican II in *Lumen Gentium* 25.[13] Moreover, if the Church had been wrong throughout the centuries on an issue of such fundamental importance as contraception, how could she maintain her claim to being the authentic interpreter of Christ's teachings?

In July of 1987, at a conference on responsible procreation, John Paul II reminded participants that the Church's consistent teaching has been vigorously expressed by Vatican II, *Humanae Vitae, Familiaris Consortio,* and *Donum Vitae.* He went on to say "The Church's teaching on contraception does not belong in the category of matter open to free discussion among theologians. Teaching the contrary amounts to leading the moral consciences of spouses into error."[14] In the words of one bishop: "The Church has not changed its teaching against contraception. What is more, the Church cannot change its teaching against contraception. Because the Church sees that teaching as based on God's moral order."[15]

Natural Family Planning

Because the Church's teaching concerning contraception has roots in the natural law, she, as would be expected, has no objection to anything that is natural. Therefore, she is an ardent supporter of a form of child-spacing or fertility regulation in marriage known as Natural Family Planning (NFP). Some have objected that NFP is "unnatural" because it requires periodic abstinence, taking the wife's body temperature, reading charts, checking mucus, and so on. In this case, however, such critics use the word "natural" to mean "spontaneous," a meaning that does not reflect the Church's mind when she uses the word in conjunction with her natural law teaching. Accordingly, what the Church means by "natural" in this context, refers to the normal functioning or proper order of things. Setting a broken humerus or using corrective lenses restores the normal functioning of the arm or the eyes. NFP is natural, not because it has any claims to spontaneity, but because it respects the order of nature. Contraception, in sundering the natural relationship between intercourse and procreation, does violence to the natural law. As Pope

John Paul II states in his Apostolic Letter, *Familiaris Consortio*: "When. . . . by means of recourse to periods of infertility, the couple respect the inseparable connection between the unitive and procreative meanings of human sexuality, they are acting as 'ministers' of God's plan and they 'benefit from' their sexuality according to the original dynamism of 'total self-giving', without manipulation or alteration."

NFP can be used, in the positive sense, to enhance the couple's chances of achieving pregnancy. In a situation where the husband has a low sperm count, for example, by combining knowledge of the time of ovulation with a period of abstinence that allows the husband to build up his sperm count, the probability for conceiving is greatly increased. On the other hand, NFP can be used, in the negative sense, in order to avoid conception. It should be noted here that NFP in the truest sense is not compatible with a "contraceptive mentality." Such a mentality, as was discussed previously, is anti-life.

Planned Parenthood's official statistician, Christopher Tietze, has reported that the effectiveness of one method of NFP — the "temperature method" — is 99%, which is higher than most contraceptives.[16] Mother Teresa, who won a Nobel Peace Prize for her work with the poor in Calcutta, reports that her NFP program in India prevented 1.1 million unwanted births in that country.[17] A study of 20,000 Hindu, Muslim, and Christian women of Calcutta who were taught NFP was reported in the *India Medical Journal*. The report stated that NFP was as successful as the Pill in avoiding unwanted pregnancies.[18] Unlike the Pill and other forms of contraception, it should be noted, NFP has no undesirable side-effects. As many practitioners of NFP have come to learn through experience, it is marriage that is the sacrament, not contraception.

The most common objection to using NFP in order to avoid conception is that it appears to be morally equivalent to using contraception. What is the difference in this case, people say, between using NFP and using contraception since the desired end is the same, namely, to avoid conception?

Apart from the issue of side-effects, which is decisive in itself, one must recognize the difference between an *end* and a *means*. Most of morality, in fact, is concerned not about ends but about means. The end, moral as it may be in itself, does not justify the employment of an immoral means. Having a child is a good end, but surely achieving that end by means of kidnapping is morally distinguishable from becoming a parent by means of loving union with one's spouse. Money may be a desirable end, but obtaining it through theft, blackmail, or extortion, as opposed to earning it justly, is the difference between immorality and morality. Virtually everyone in the history of moral philosophy recognizes the validity of this distinction. Contraception violates the order established in nature by God between intercourse and procreation.

Also, there is a profound difference between an immoral act and no act at all. This difference is not only metaphysical (between being and nonbeing), but can be felt personally and intensely on a psychological level. Suppose, for example, an engaged couple is preparing its list of wedding guests. The couple wants some people to come and others not to come. The traditional approach is to invite those whom you want to be your guests, and not invite those whom you do not. But let us imagine that this particular couple, instead of simply not inviting certain people, sends them a disinvitation: "Dear John and Mary: We are getting married, but we do not want you to come to our wedding. Our ushers have been instructed to escort you to the parking lot if you dare show up. Your presence is not wanted. Stay away. We do not want to see you."

It is not difficult to appreciate the difference in impact on John's and Mary's feelings that receiving such a "disinvitation" would have, as compared with their not receiving an invitation. Sending out such a disinvitation could very well ruin whatever vestige of friendship existed between the two parties. The difference between the disinvitation and no invitation is the difference between insult and etiquette, contempt and civility. It is one thing not to invite a person; it is quite another to explain to him that his presence is unwanted.

Using contraception is like sending a disinvitation to God. It is like telling God that He should not show up, that His creative act is not only unwanted, but disrespected. But abstaining from intercourse as part of NFP does not send any such message. By refraining from intercourse at a time when a couple does not want to conceive sends an altogether different and more tacit message: "We do not invite or invoke your creative act at this time, but we will not insult you by profaning the means you have established to inititate new life by exploiting it for our own purposes while disinviting your presence through contraception. We will abstain rather than profane."

Another common objection to the Church's promotion of NFP and rejection of contraception is that it represents a beautiful "ideal," but it is not very practical for most married couples. But NFP has proven to be eminently practical wherever it has been used, whereas the "ideals" that contraception promoters envisioned, such as less sexual anxiety, happier marriages, fewer divorces, and better rapport between parents and children, have proven to be decidedly impractical and unrealistic.

Among married couples who practice NFP, divorce is rare. Josef Rötzer, M. D., author of a sympto-thermal method, reports not a single divorce or abortion among 1,400 married couples who used NFP. John Kippley, founder of the Couple to Couple League, reports a 1.3% divorce rate among married couple who teach NFP.[19]

The contraception debate is not between an out-dated Church whose ideals are unrealistic and a modern, secular world that has no ideals but is hard-nosed and realistic. The debate is between the Church, whose ideals are realistic (in the sense that they can, with effort, be realized) and a world whose ideals are not. Contraception advocates are not without ideals. It is simply that their ideals cannot be realized through the contraceptive means that they propose. To believe that contraception will bring about a greater two-in-one-flesh intimacy is to believe in an impossibility.

An ideal may be difficult, but it should not be dismissed simply because it is an ideal. The "ideal" for each hole in golf is to make par (that is to say, the "realistic" or "reasonable" ideal, rather than the improbable ideal of making a hole-in-one on each tee-shot). In fact, this is a minimal ideal. Amateur golfers and the legion of struggling recreational performers known as "duffers," often find this ideal hard to fulfill. Yet no golfer protests that golf is an unrealistic game and that par should be whatever number of strokes it takes for a player to complete a hole. The "ideal" is necessary to give the game its structure, meaning, and direction. With no ideal to realize, there can never be any sense of fulfillment.

It is precisely because the Church's teaching is based on the natural law that her ideals are both realistic and realizable. By contrast, the ideals of the world are often based on dreams that have no relationship with either nature or the natural law. Such dreams are fundamentally unrealistic.

Personalism

Because man is ordered to God, the separation of the marital act from procreation also separates man as a person from God. Neither the personal nor the spiritual can be entirely divorced from the physical. Contraception, in separating the sex act from life, inevitably separates, at least to some degree, the sexual being from the author of life. Spiritual contraception is a predictable consequence of physical contraception. To erect a barrier against God's creative act is inseparable from becoming alienated from God in other ways. The contraceptive barrier against reality is also a barrier against truth. According to one theologian, "God, through His Church, both denounces contraception and proffers the graces to regulate the size of one's family by continence. Disbelief in the one truth implies disbelief in the other."[20] The contraceptive act that excludes God may also exclude His grace.

Continence can be a greater expression of love than contraceptive sex. When husband and wife decide, with good reason, to forego the marital act rather than use contraception, they honor the personal wholeness that sexual union implies. It is better that they not use sex to express their love than to misuse it. A married couple honors the wholeness of the marital act in two ways only: 1) positively, by expressing it in its natural wholeness and integrity; 2) negatively, by not expressing it at all, rather than defiling it by expressing it in a vitiated way. The same can be said about telling the truth. One may tell the truth or not say anything at all. But it is the falsified truth, the lie, which is morally objectionable.

The fact that physical contraception leads to spiritual contraception is perhaps nowhere better evidenced than in what has been referred to as the current "Condom Generation." The condom has become a metaphor for isolation, not only from new life and sexually transmitted diseases, but from any intrusion or penetration from the outside world, including truth, love, and grace. A university student has explained the matter simply and directly: "We are the condom generation. We have learned to protect ourselves against intrusion, mental, auditory, physical, emotional. Don't try the shock treatment, it will have the opposite effect from what you hope."[21]

Victims of the Condom Generation distrust everything that is not part of themselves. Given time, when they realize that there is no justification for trusting themselves and no one else, they learn to distrust themselves as well. The spiritual contraception that physical contraception engenders makes it exceedingly difficult to communicate to those who are practicing contraception the truth about the alienating effect their practice has on them.

The Church's teaching on contraception is based on the natural law, incorporates the sacramental character of marriage, honors the dignity of the marital act, and affirms the sacredness of new human life. In addition, it recognizes man's nature as a *person*, that is, an embodied, engendered, being-in-the-world, who lives and develops through knowledge and love.

A person is an individual, unique and unrepeatable; but a person is, at the same time, communal and capable of profound interpersonal relationships. In referring to the personalistic implications of marriage, the most common and fundamental form of human community, John Paul states that "this conjugal communion sinks roots in the natural complementarity that exists between man and woman and is nurtured through the personal willingness of the spouses to share their entire life project, what they have and what they are. For this reason, such communion is the fruit and sign of a profoundly human need."[22]

Contraception, as John Paul II has pointed out on many occasions, contradicts the "innate language that expresses the total reciprocal self-giving of husband and wife."[23] In a verbal lie, the word contradicts what one knows to be the case. In a bodily lie, the body's expression (the language of the body) contradicts the meaning the person ascribes to that bodily expression. When Judas gave Christ a kiss, he did not intend it to mean friendship, which a kiss signifies naturally, but to indicate betrayal. His kiss was a lie. He did not intend it to mean what it means in the natural language of the body. Contraceptive intercourse is a lie on a deeply personal level because, on the one hand, intercourse symbolizes the total giving of the partners to each other, whereas contraception, on the other hand, is their willful negation of each other's procreative potential.

As a *person*, a human being is not simply a body or simply a spirit, but an embodied spirit. Sexuality, therefore, is not merely biological. To allege that contraception negates only the biological dimension, leaving the partners free to have sex with each other on a more spiritual level, is to do violence to the integrity of the person. Sexuality is diffused throughout the whole of one's personality. When husband and wife share the marital act, they express love to each other as incarnate persons, not as either animals or angels. Man is a person. Contraception contradicts his integrity and wholeness as a person.

The possibility that the marriage act can produce a child, a new image of God, gives husband and wife a dimension that clearly transcends their individualities. Recognition of this *supra-personal* dimension elicits a sense of wonder and privilege, what one might call *awe*. An American woman reported that she and her husband were able to experience "awe" once they abandoned contraception and allowed God to re-enter their conjugal relationship.[24] An Australian woman reports this same sense of "awe" when she and her husband honor God's creative presence.[25] Finally, a Pulitzer Prize winning novelist makes essentially the same point that if such "awe" is not experienced between the sexes, their union is reduced to a mere transaction. To exclude the procreative possibility is not only to invite lust and power, he maintains, but to abandon that world of love in which God is the supreme master.[26]

As a person, one lives, not by lust, but by love. Love, which is the promotion of the good of another, proceeds from the wholeness of the loving person. True love between spouses is a synthesis of two wholes, two persons in one flesh. Lust is fragmentary. It is a synthesis between fragments, between appetite and that part of the other that arouses the appetite. Lust aims at the disintegration of personality, a direction that is essentially meaningless. Lust is also chained to necessity, whereas love is always given in an atmosphere of freedom. Contraception prevents love from being truly whole. Because of its fragmentary propensities, it is highly compatible with lust.

Referring to the incarnate love that husband and wife freely share with one another, Pope Paul VI writes:

> This love is of the senses and of the spirit at the same time. It is not, then, merely a question of natural instinct or emotional drive. It is also and above all, an act of free will, whose dynamism ensures that not only does it endure through the joys and sorrows of daily life, but also that it grows, so that husband and wife becomes in a way, one heart and one soul, and together attain their human fulfillment.[27]

For John Paul II, that which "constitutes the essential evil of the contraceptive act" is the way it violates the interior order of conjugal union, an order that is rooted in the very order of the person.[28]

The Church teaches that the spouses minister the sacrament of marriage to each other. It is, therefore, most fitting that as they express, in sexual union, that mysterious language of their bodies, they do so in all truth that is proper to it.

Conclusion

Humanae Vitae affirms the Church's consistent and historical teaching that there is an "inseparable connection, willed by God and unable to be broken by man on his own initiative, between the two meanings of the conjugal act: the unitive and the procreative."[29]

This teaching is not a mere "ideal" for those who find contraception to be more "realistic." It is eminently practicable, as attested by the great successes reported throughout the world by couples who practice Natural Family Planning. Moreover, because NFP honors the personal wholeness of its practitioners, it accords with the nature and dignity of their incarnate humanity.

Church teaching concerning NFP recognizes the priority that the *person* has over *pleasure*, that *love* has over *appetite*, and that *generosity* has over *selfishness*.

Those married couples who honor the unitive and procreative meanings of the sexual act in their lives are in a most favorable position to grow closer to each other without separating themselves from God. They understand that the dignity of procreation and the sacredness of new life bear a direct relation to Christ, who instituted marriage, and God the Father, who creates new life.

A good marriage is the basis for a good family. Since the family remains the fundamental unit of society, a good marriage plays an immense and indispensable role in providing essential benefits for society. The future of humanity passes through the husbands and wives whose invocations of life confer upon them the status of fathers and mothers. The quality of today's marriage is crucial to the quality of life for the next generation.

The Church's teaching concerning marriage and contraception is directed to the home, but its implications are far-reaching, both in time and in space. One of the greatest disappointments the Church has experienced in the second half of the twentieth century is not so much the informed dissent from and conscientious rejection of *Humanae Vitae*, but in so many Catholics turning a blind eye and a deaf ear to its liberating message. It is the truth, not the capacity to dismiss Church teaching, that makes people truly free. The Promethean gesture is self-defeating. God is man's supreme benefactor and the Church is his most reliable teacher. The Church shines a light that reveals the holiness of marriage, the value of the family, and the inviolability of human life. She is also a channel of grace that helps make the truth livable, and a community of helpmates who assist in making them shareable. Her truths are the truths that will enable husbands and wives to find the freedom they need in order to love each other as God wills, and to raise children who will take their rightful places in the world and continue the work of renewing the face of the earth.

Endnotes

[1] Thomas Aquinas, *Summa Theologica*, I, 1,1.

[2] Thomas Aquinas, *Summa Contra Gentiles*, I, 4.

[3] Janet E. Smith, "Humanae Vitae: A Hidden Treasure," *The British Columbia Catholic*, Nov. 7, 1993. Dr. Smith is the author of a major study on Pope Paul VI's encyclical on contraception — *Humanae Vitae: A Generation Later* (Washiington, D.C.: Catholic University of America Press, 1991). She is also the editor of *Why Humanae Vitae Was Right: A Reader* (San Francisco, CA: Ignatius Press, 1993).

[4]Blanca Reilly, "Gender Politics at the U. N.," *Crisis*, June 1995, p. 10.

[5]*Exodus* 3: 05: "Take off your shoes, for the place on which you stand is holy ground."

[6]Germain Grisez, Joseph Boyle, John Finnis, and William E. May, "'Every Marital Act Ought To Be Open To New Life': Toward A Clearer Understanding," *The Thomist*, 52, 3, July, 1988, pp. 365-426. Here the authors develop and explain in great detail the "contralife" implications of contraception.

[7]Pope John Paul II, in his "Theology of the Body" speaks extensively of the "gift of self" that husband and wife bring to their marriage. See John Paul II, *Original Unity of Man and Woman: Catechesis on the Book of Genesis* (Boston, MA: Daughters of St. Paul, 1981).

[8]Pope Paul VI, *Humanae Vitae*, sec. 12.

[9]*Ibid.*, sec. 14, See also *Catechism of the Catholic Church* (Ottawa, ON: Canadian Conference of Catholic Bishops, 1992), section 2370, p. 483.

[10]Sigmund Freud, *A General Introduction to Psycho-Analysis*, trans. by Joan Riviere (New York, NY: Liverwright, 1935), p. 277.

[11]"Minority Papal Commission Report," *The Catholic Case for Contraception*, Daniel Callahan (ed.), (London, England: Collier-Macmillan, 1969), p. 179.

[12]Ronald Lawler, Joseph Boyle, and William E. May, *Catholic Sexual Ethics* (Huntington, IN: Our Sunday Visitor, 1985), p. 156. See also John Paul II, *Familiaris Consortio*, sec. 29.

[13]John C. Ford, S.J., and Germain Grisez, "Contraception and the Infallibility of the Ordinary Magisterium," *Theological Studies*, June 1978, Vol. 39, No. 2, pp. 258-312.

[14]John Paul II, "The Church's teaching on contraception is not a matter for free discussion among theologians," *L'Osservatore Romano*, July 6, 1987.

[15]Archbishop John F. Whealon of Hartford, CT, *The Hartford Catholic Transcript*, Feb. 28, 1980.

[16]Herbert F. Smith, S.J., "The Proliferation of Population Problems," *Why Humanae Vitae Was Right*, Janet E. Smith (ed.), (San Francisco, CA: Ignatius Press, 1993). p. 399.

[17]"The Billings Ovulation Method of Birth Regulation," (World Organization Ovulation Method Billings, undated flyer), p. 1.

[18]Jon Hunt, "Doctor defends the natural method," *Birmingham Post* (England).

[19]Janet E. Smith, *op. cit. 1993*, p. 432. John Kippley, *The Catholic Dossier, op. cit.*, p. 48.

[20]Paul Quay, "Contraception and Conjugal Love," Janet E. Smith (ed.), *op. cit. 1993*, p. 43.

[21]Professor Janine Langan made this point in her opening address at the Second Panamerican Conference on Family and Education, Toronto, ON, May 27, 1996. See also Janine Langan, *The Catholic Register*, Nov. 18, 1996.

[22]*Familiaris Consortio*, sec. 19.

[23]*Ibid.*

[24]*National Catholic Register,*Oct. 11, 1987.

[25]Melinda Reist, *The Pill and Liberation Methodology* (Stafford, VA: American Life League, 1992), p. 10.

[26]Norman Mailer, *The Prisoner of Sex* (Boston, MA: Little, Brown & Co., 1971), pp. 173-74.

[27]*Humanae Vitae*, sec. 9.

[28]John Paul II, *Reflections of Humanae Vitae* (Boston, MA: Daughters of St. Paul, 1984), p. 33.

[29]*Humanae Vitae*, sec. 12. For an excellent presentation and analysis of this encyclical, see Janet E. Smith, *Humanae Vitae: A Generation Later* (Washington, DC: The Catholic University of America Press, 1991), chapters 3-5. Her translation, direct from Latin to English, including several pages of commentary, is also available from New Hope Publications, New Hope, KY, 270-325-3061.

Eternal Values

In the bright mid-morning sun,
The porch-light faintly glimmers;
Faithful to a function
Made redundant by the dawn.

Not long ago it served:
Proudly as a beacon,
Gently as a glow reserved
For all returning home.

It's role now obsolete,
Anachronistically,
It lingers in defeat,
Devoid of point or purpose.

Soon enough the night
Will wrap the world in darkness
And once again this vesicle of light
Will radiate its glory.

— by Donald DeMarco

"DeMarco never disappoints, and this treatment of the faulty reasoning behind man's fascination with contraception is more than a new look at an age-old problem. We go with DeMarco on an investigative chase. He leads the way in hot pursuit of the case of the dying human race. He unfolds the clues that expose man's ability to deny or accept God's love.

"We travel down the dark alleys of lust, self-centered imagery and ultimate rejection of the value of the human person. We watch man suffer, we see him resist the soft embrace of the Lord, and we see him fail to achieve his false freedom while left laying in the abyss caused by materialism and loneliness.

"Detective DeMarco reveals the other trail of clues—the story of the human being who tries to understand the design of nature, and ultimately succeeds because he pursues truth and takes the road less traveled. DeMarco will challenge every reader to follow the signs, think about the consequences and sort out the differences between instant gratification and long-term satisfaction. *New Perspectives* is a book for everyone who has ever wondered why society seems so dead set on destroying itself."

—Judie Brown, President
American Life League

"Dr. Donald DeMarco's *New Perspectives on Contraception* is a comprehensive and thought-provoking look into the contraceptive mentality of our society. It is the reader who will triumph if this book is carefully read, because Dr. DeMarco leads one to the wise conclusion that 'UnNatural Family Planning,' as he calls it, is far from the correct answer to today's many challenges, not the least of which is infertility."

—Sue & Kay Ek
Billings Ovulation Method-USA

"Don DeMarco's latest book shows that to be against birth control is far from an outdated position. He supports his position within the best scientific, sociological, and philosophical wisdom available, and presents it in common sense readable fashion. Our society does not have a problem of being obsessed with sex. On the contrary, it is afraid of sex. By treating this gift so superficially, it has failed to truly encounter it and appreciate its significance. *New Perspectives on Contraception* goes a long way toward solving this problem, and I strongly recommend it to everyone in pastoral ministry, to all in the pro-life movement, and to anyone who has the courage to reexamine his or her views on the subject."

—Fr. Frank Pavone
National Director, Priests for Life